Lupus:
In the Jaws
of the Wolf

Lupus:
In the Jaws
of the Wolf

A Physician's Personal Guide
to Living with Lupus

NIRANJANA PARTHASARATHI, M.D.

Lupus: In the Jaws of the Wolf
A Physician's Personal Guide to Living with Lupus

Niranjana Parthasarathi, M.D.

Published by Niranjana Parthasarathi, M.D.

ISBN: 979-8-218-07826-3

Library of Congress Control Number: 2023900281

Disclaimer: The information contained herein is for educational purposes only and is the result of years of practice and experience by the author. However, it is not a substitute for evaluation and treatment by a medical doctor and is not intended to be a substitute for professional medical advice. The reader should always consult with his or her physician to determine the appropriateness of the information for his or her own medical situation and treatment plan. Reading this book does not constitute a physician-patient relationship. Products or services mentioned in this book are for reference purposes only. The author does not receive referral compensation of any kind.

Dedicated to my husband and companion,
Dan Fitzsimmons, in appreciation
of his love and support.

Contents

Introduction

Those confronting lupus and those who love us may feel bittersweet emotions in reading this lovely, hopeful quote from the poet Mary Oliver. Like some other chronic illnesses, life with lupus, derived from the Latin for "wolf," is complex and unpredictable. It is far more demanding than those unaffected can understand. Lupus, or systemic lupus erythematosus (SLE), causes overwhelming, life-altering fatigue and bodily pain. It can be life-threatening due to organ injury. Both the severity and progression of the disease vary over time, making it a challenging, inescapable, and unwanted companion.

I am a lupus patient and an internal medicine physician. I was a professor of clinical medicine at the University of

Cincinnati College of Medicine for twenty years until becoming disabled by lupus at age fifty. My purpose with this guide is to share knowledge, insights, and suggestions from my thirty-seven-year history of cohabiting with the "wolf," enduring multiple organ complications, and coming to terms with the disease. A good quality of life with lupus is truly possible despite the many challenges, discouragement, and despair that can occur.

In addition to our physical health, lupus attacks our very core and affects every aspect of our lives. Relationships with family and friends are impacted, and those closest to us suffer and sacrifice as our illness alters their lives, too. Our ability to work and maintain our independence is often disrupted, with financial tensions resulting. Interests and hobbies are often lost, as poor energy levels constrain us. The fluctuating symptoms make honoring commitments very difficult.

My hope is to encourage and inspire those of you afflicted with the "cruel mystery," as the Lupus Foundation calls it. I use the wolf motif throughout, as it's a vivid symbol of lupus. Rather than viewing it as our enemy, we must learn to coexist with it. Living with lupus presents an opportunity for personal growth and the development of resilience. Acceptance, gratitude, and a deep appreciation of each moment and breath can result if we are open to them.

Lupus is an incurable but treatable autoimmune disease in which the immune system, which normally protects us from infections or incipient cancer, instead attacks the body. It can be either localized or involve the whole body, as in the case of SLE. This is the most common and severe form of lupus and will be my focus. The highest estimated prevalence of lupus worldwide is in North America, with 240 cases per 100,000 people. The disease is likely underdiagnosed,[1] and the Lupus Foundation of America estimates that about 1.5 million adults in the U.S. currently suffer from SLE.

Estrogen plays a role in triggering the disease, so over 90 percent of the affected are women. However, men tend to have more severe illness. It typically strikes women in their childbearing years, though children and teens are also sometimes afflicted. White Caucasians can develop severe lupus, but the condition is more prevalent and severe in nonwhite individuals. It is estimated to strike African Americans more than twice as often as whites. It is believed to originate from a genetic predisposition coupled with an infectious trigger. Both rheumatoid arthritis and lupus share a common genetic predisposition.[2] Thus, both are seen in some families.

Early symptoms are variable and include constitutional (bodily) symptoms such as fatigue, fevers, headaches, and malaise, or a flu-like feeling. Musculoskeletal symptoms mainly involve muscles and joints, though other connective tissue, such as tendons, can also be affected. These include muscle pain, joint pain, and joint swelling, known as arthritis. Mucocutaneous manifestations affect mucous membranes, the tissue lining your body cavities, and skin. Painless mouth ulcers, which are peculiar to lupus, and skin rashes are the most common of these signs. The "butterfly" or malar facial lupus rash occurs in many patients. Rashes and mouth ulcers are often triggered by ultraviolet radiation from the sun or other sources.

More severe lupus can attack any organ and system in the body with varying manifestations. Several studies show that 30 to 50 percent of patients have developed organ damage within ten years of illness. The early symptoms of the disease can be very vague, making the diagnosis difficult. The symptoms, signs (objective findings on examination), and organ involvement change unpredictably over time. The wolf is an appropriate symbol for the disease, as it can viciously wreak havoc upon lupus patients.

The most used diagnostic criteria were developed in 2019 by the American College of Rheumatology. These defining benchmarks and medical knowledge of the disease continue to develop. They are numerous and complex and include the presence of specific autoantibodies, which are antibodies directed against oneself. Arthritis, rashes, kidney disease, and blood disorders are other possible diagnostic manifestations. Certain neurologic and psychiatric conditions and inflammation around the heart or lungs can also help to confirm lupus.

Rarely, there is a remission of the illness, but for most, the symptoms wax and wane over time. A British study of about

500 lupus patients found that 14.5 percent achieved remission lasting at least three years, though only 4 percent remained in remission at ten years.[3] Relapses occurred even after ten years, and those with major organ disease were far less likely to enjoy a respite. Even a long remission does not mean we are free of the wolf's grasp.

Most of us lupus "warriors" will have a mild disease, so we should remain calm upon receiving the diagnosis. Remember that the manifestations are highly inconsistent. My severe, multi-organ disease course is not representative, though lupus can be extremely debilitating. Flares, or worsening symptoms that can involve organ injury, can be triggered by both physical and emotional stress. The evolution in understanding and treatments has improved prognosis over the past few decades. But there is still much unknown, and tragically, some still die prematurely of the disease.

Excellent self-care can help prevent the disease from becoming severe and disabling, and I will address these measures in detail later. We should avoid catastrophizing and imagining the worst-case scenarios. As Bismarck noted, "Life is like being at the dentist. We always think that the worst is yet to come, and yet it is over already!"

Despite evidence to the contrary, we humans tend to believe we have a reasonable degree of control over our health. Even healthcare workers, who witness the randomness of illness, fall prey to this. Although we know that good habits increase the odds of longevity, some with healthy habits die young, while a few who abuse their bodies live to a ripe old age. In my early years with lupus, I convinced myself that it was controllable. Over time, I realized I could only moderate its consequences and learn to cope with it better.

A lack of understanding is universal with lupus, like other "invisible" illnesses, and further complicates our lives. Our often-normal outward appearance can contradict how we feel, leading some to call SLE the "liar's disease." The exhaustion, pain, and other symptoms are often hidden. Some other chronic conditions, including other autoimmune diseases, multiple sclerosis, ME/CFS (myalgic encephalomyelitis/chronic fatigue syndrome), chronic Lyme disease, and long COVID, can also be met with skepticism due to the normal appearance of the patient.

Misconceptions about chronic illness have likely always existed and complicated the lives of those affected. In the novels of eighteenth-century novelist Jane Austen, for example, there is often a female character who is chronically ill and unable to join the others on romps around the countryside. This character was mocked and viewed as hypochondriacal, revealing a lack of empathy and "ableism" or discrimination in favor of the "able-bodied." We see these attitudes persisting today, most recently in the disbelief long COVID patients sometimes experience.

I will first briefly relate the story of my life with lupus beginning with some childhood background. My husband, Dan, has contributed a few observations to provide a loved one's perspective. Then, some healthcare inequities impacting those of us with lupus and other chronic diseases will be described. Detailed practical management and lifestyle measures to help maintain health will follow. As we warriors can be medically complex and require several specialists, we must be knowledgeable and very involved in our care. Finally, I will address coping with the stress and uncertainty of chronic illness.

Finding and maintaining a sense of purpose in the midst of chronic illness can be difficult. For us warriors, joining support groups and aiding one another can provide an uplifting goal. If my account helps my fellow patients, my struggles with lupus become more meaningful.

PART ONE

In the Jaws of the Wolf

The Wolf Lies in Wait

"You think your pain and heartbreak are unprecedented in the world, but then you read."

– James Baldwin

As an Indian American growing up in northern Virginia just after the civil rights movement, my childhood was hardly a typical one. We came to the U.S. when I was two years old. My parents were loving but made it clear that we were Indian and expected to behave traditionally, as we were truly just temporary visitors to the United States. I realized over time that this was my father's rationalization for taking a job at the World Bank on an international organization employee visa. His cultural pride and perhaps defensiveness about his heritage were understandable. After all, the British colonization of India ended relatively recently, in 1947.

So, unlike the typical immigrant tendency to rapidly assimilate into the culture of their new homeland, my parents, like many other South Asians, raised their children as they were reared. They ignored the fact that social mores and conventions were changing in their countries of origin. The ensuing "culture clash" my parents foisted upon us made our lives more difficult, adding to the subtle but different treatment from some of our predominantly white classmates. While we did have friends, my older brother and I occasionally suffered feelings of isolation and alienation.

By middle school, I realized that even some of the most "American" looking of my classmates were afflicted by this and that it's part of being human. Obviously, my skin color would mark me as a "foreigner" for the rest of my life, a harsh reality. My father continued fantasizing about returning to and dying in his homeland until the end. Only his love for his children and grandchildren prevented him from doing so.

In our travels to India every other summer, I first became aware of the depth of agony in the world as we were inundated with beggars in the cities. The scale of misery was such that even as a relatively young child, I recall feeling depressed and anxious to return home, where we were insulated from poverty. I was a voracious reader and enjoyed literature from around the world. The pivotal moment that led me to go into medicine was reading *The Plague* by Albert Camus in high school, which convinced me that fighting injustice and suffering should be my life's work. As I lacked the personality, charisma, or confidence to achieve these goals on a larger scale, I felt drawn to medicine.

Reading increased my awareness of the many problems in our world. It was crucial to my sensitivity and ability to cope with the tragedies I later witnessed in healthcare. This may explain why many medical schools have increasingly adopted literature into their curricula and why undergraduate arts majors are welcomed.

Like many families, mine was somewhat dysfunctional, with highly traditional and incompatible parents joined by arranged marriage. My father was a deeply loving and generous person. However, he was also volatile, with an unpredictable temper triggered at times by minor infractions. It was directed towards all of us, especially my mother, and it made me feel at times that he saw us as the obstacles to his perfectionism. As is often the case with people who lash out, he was a very wounded individual. I knew only vaguely that his childhood was traumatic.

The eldest of seven children, my father was sent off at age nine to live with various relatives and family friends due to his parents' poverty. Only after his death did I learn from a cousin that the extended family knew that my poor father had been badly abused during some of these years. I wasn't surprised, though he refused to ever acknowledge there was a problem.

He was a brilliant high achiever who got a master's degree by age eighteen and began supporting the entire family of nine. His father was too irresponsible to work regularly as a journalist and quit when the whim seized him.

My mother's family, in contrast, was happy and solidly middle-class. My maternal grandmother was among the few matriarchs I've seen in Indian culture. She was a strong, capable woman, and my grandfather was placid and respectful of her. Amma, my mother, took after her father and is a sweet, kind person. She is a very devout Hindu and dependent, lacking self-confidence. Living with my father from age twenty-one would certainly diminish even the most self-possessed person, as he was critical and sometimes verbally abusive.

At age nine, I became my mother's confidant as she puzzled unhappily over what drove dad's irascible behavior. I learned early in life that it was my job to take care of my mother, and as I matured, I often challenged my father when he was behaving unkindly. It was the whole family's job to "protect" my parents, as anything that upset my father led him to lose his temper. Culturally, counseling or the idea of sharing one's problems was unacceptable, so neither sought the psychological help that could have benefited them. Amma sharing her sorrow with me reflected how completely trapped she felt.

My mother tried to inculcate a patriarchal worldview in me, as she was annoyed by my habit of questioning everything.

She felt only males had the right to do so, while females had to be endlessly patient and tolerant—which made no sense to me. This doubtlessly helped her cope with living with my father. She worried that if I didn't mold myself into a compliant person, I would "end up divorced like my aunt!" Early on, I decided this blatant misogyny was wrong and ignored it, later ending up divorced as she predicted!

My father told me in high school that I didn't have to work and could have a "comfortable, easier life" like Amma and my aunt via an arranged marriage. I had no interest whatsoever in Appa's idea of marrying me off, and felt strongly about the importance of contributing to this troubled world. I also knew firsthand the potential indignity of financial dependency.

My childhood travel to India made me consider moving there to practice medicine, as the need is overwhelming. During college, volunteering at a free clinic and a state psychiatric hospital showed me the depth of deprivation in our own country, too. The U.S. is the only home I have known, and I decided to pursue indigent care right here. The sexism experienced during visits to India was even worse than in the United States. Indian women physicians in that era were expected to become gynecologists or pediatricians.

Early emotional wounds undoubtedly influenced my impulse towards a healing profession, something others in healthcare have experienced. Perhaps the unfulfilled wish to heal one's family leads to a compulsion to heal the world.

Medicine provides the hope of a better outcome and relief of distress we could not achieve at home. It has been observed that people choose their specialty based on where their personal need lies. We want to help others who share our vulnerabilities and be better equipped to deal with our own.

I lacked the degree of introspection necessary to heal myself emotionally in young adulthood. Like many who choose a demanding profession, I was too busy for self-analysis. Distraction was perhaps the intent, on some level. Eventually, in my thirties, I recognized the need to get counseling when considering parenthood. I wanted to ensure that I would escape some of the patterns of my family and minimize trauma for my child.

Facing the Wolf

"Life . . . was a series of losses. It was other things too, better things, but the losses were as solid and dependable as the earth itself."

– Ann Patchett

The first time I heard of lupus was when I was twenty-three and a second-year medical student. The professor excitedly described it as the "most fascinating of diseases," as it can manifest in myriad ways, potentially affecting any part of the body. I thought it sounded absolutely awful, unsuspecting that I would soon become a "fascinoma," or an interesting case, myself! Looking back on it now, I can laugh at the irony of his comment.

Later that year, I developed symptoms of joint pain, swelling, and morning stiffness in the fingers. When my symptoms lasted for over a month, I became concerned. My friends joked that I was suffering "medical student-itis," as medical students are notorious for imagining the worst while learning the infinite ways our bodies can malfunction. We were awestruck by the usual precision of our body's intricate mechanisms.

As my symptoms worsened, I turned to the dean of the medical school, who referred me to a rheumatologist or specialist in lupus, other autoimmune diseases, and arthritis. His initial diagnosis was that I likely had rheumatoid arthritis, which two family members on my father's side also had. My uncle suffered with severe, deforming rheumatoid arthritis and died in his early sixties of complications of the disease.

The rheumatologist suggested I might wish to consider a less physically demanding field after medical school, such as psychiatry or radiology, given the diagnosis. I received symptomatic treatment with the anti-inflammatory naproxen, which was recommended then. I improved quickly and gave it very little thought, as I was focused on learning the vast amount of material that medical students must master.

During my third year of medical school in the 1980s, I began clinical rotations in the hospital. This involved, on average, spending every fourth night night at the hospital. We worked the next day, often nearly thirty-six hours at a stretch. We students considered ourselves lucky if we could get a few hours of sleep, and this sleep deficit occasionally triggered mild joint symptoms for me. I was fatigued, but so were all my classmates. For most of the third year of medical school, we spent at least eighty to one hundred hours a week in the hospital. The thrill and stimulation of hospital work more than compensated for the workload.

After a stressful start to the year, I became more comfortable with hospital duties. Though I found the basic sciences interesting, it wasn't until I could utilize my knowledge to take care of people that I fell in love with the science and art of medicine. I thrived in the atmosphere of the university medical center, where lectures and case discussions supplemented learning by assisting in patient care.

One morning, I awoke with a red, hot, swollen wrist and pink eyes and went to the student health center. The doctor there sent me to a faculty rheumatologist, who kindly saw me immediately. He injected my wrist with steroids and ordered lab testing. I had also been having a mild chronic dry cough. The next day, I bumped into my new rheumatologist in the hospital cafeteria, and he immediately examined my wrist, gratified to see the excellent response to his injection.

This was long before patient privacy was considered, and embarrassed, I chided him for publicly discussing my condition. I already felt the need to appear invulnerable, even as a medical student. This was the first episode in a long pattern of behavior that displayed the avoidance of my illness. After all, if I concealed it and no one knew, there was no problem, right? Wrong.

A few days later, my doctor informed me that I had lupus based on my lab test results. I was terrified and broke down in tears, much to his surprise. My reaction was based both on knowledge of the disease's gravity and personal experience. The young woman who was my dormitory roommate in my first year of medical school had recently died of lupus complications during her obstetrics and gynecology internship. As she was a third-year student spending all her time in the hospital or library, I rarely saw her. I shared her death with him, and he assured me the disease was treatable.

My *Cecil Textbook of Medicine* informed me that those with lupus need more rest than most. There was little information in that era regarding lifestyle measures to mitigate the disease. Over the decades, I learned more about what could help through my reading, physicians' advice, and trial and error.

To further evaluate the mild cough I'd been having, lung function tests were done. They revealed a very mild decreased oxygen uptake in my tiny airways or lung interstitium. This was possibly due to autoimmune injury to the air sacs, causing mild scarring.

Initially, I coped with the diagnosis poorly and was in denial, focusing on my studies. I was determined not to allow lupus to interfere with my plans. I told only my family and a few close friends about it. A part of me feared dying young, but I knew that most with lupus have a mild illness. The diagnosis saddened me, as I had lost what we all consider to be essential in life: good health. Over the decades, I occasionally reflect on feeling unwell for almost all my adult life and how wonderful it would be to experience feeling fine for even one day.

The delusion of the invincibility of youth helped me suppress my fears and focus on my life's work. There was likely an element of magical thinking, which led me to buy into the myth in the medical community of superhuman capacity. After all, if I were focusing on healing others, surely, I would remain healthy. Over the decades, I learned of many cases in which physicians overlooked their own health problems, sometimes resulting in severe illness or death.

Having recently begun helping to care for patients, I was utterly fascinated by the process of diagnosing and treating illness. I was also sometimes intimidated by my first experience working in this setting. I could see that I was healthier than my hospitalized patients, whom I reasoned needed care far more than I did.

Denial is a natural response many of us have upon receiving a serious diagnosis, but a few factors aggravated this in my case. First was the culture of medicine, which encouraged, fostered, and expected dedication to patient care above all else. The second was my parents' response to bad health news, reinforcing my tendency toward avoidance as the simplest response. Interestingly, among some Hindus, there is a sense of shame about illness, perhaps because it is viewed as the result of terrible inherited karma by the individual and their parents.

In hindsight, I wonder if there wasn't an element of self-destructiveness in continuing to plunge myself into an incredibly physically and psychologically demanding career. Was my self-preservation instinct impaired? Knowing that a fellow student died at thirty, wouldn't it have made sense for me to reconsider my chosen path? Was my life of no value unless I was serving others, and was taking care of others more important than taking care of myself?

These questions still haunt me as I consider the severe flare that was to appear decades later. Perhaps we women are raised to be too self-sacrificing and nurturing of others, at times to our detriment. Maybe an element of "survivor's guilt" in those of us from developing countries played a role. Staring grinding poverty in the face drove me to feel I must try to help heal the world. Perhaps surprisingly, my optimistic temperament persists, which has both helped and hurt me over the years. My sense of humor and love of laughter also sustain me. Despite lupus, I consider myself happy and fortunate overall.

We patients should never fall into the trap of blaming ourselves for our illness, though our families sometimes do. My mother and brother are still certain that my medical work "caused" my illness, for example. They'd like to think I'm in more control of it than is realistic. This may also be a defense mechanism, as it protects one from the reality that catastrophic illness can suddenly strike anyone. Those with lupus simply have the misfortune of having a chronic disease that makes our lives far more unpredictable than most.

This is a lesson I'm still absorbing, as letting go of the past is still occasionally difficult. Despite knowing the eventual consequences I will share later, I still have no regrets. In my practice, I learned that most people dislike their jobs and find them unfulfilling. I was able to work full-time for thirty years, including medical school, pursuing my passion in life—something many people never experience.

* * *

In retrospect, I realized that my first signs and symptoms of lupus began in high school. I had mild fatigue and recurrent problems with severe red eyes, probably due to autoimmune inflammation. My family belonged to a health maintenance organization in Washington, D.C., and routine screening for syphilis was done on all patients in those days, as the 1970s were the era of "free love" and rampant sexually transmitted infections. One day, not long after a family trip to India, my father received a phone call from the public health department stating that I needed testing for possible venereal disease, which he misheard as "malarial disease."

I was shocked when we arrived at the health department and realized what they were testing for, as I was a skinny, bespectacled, awkward fourteen-year-old who'd never had a boyfriend, much less sex! On the way home, I told my father, "There must be some mistake—I haven't done anything!" An economist with no medical training, my dad chuckled in response and said that I must have picked it up from the school toilets. The lab confirmed that the initial test was a false positive. It reflected the presence of an autoantibody or antibody directed against me, cross-reacting with the syphilis screening test. This false positive RPR (rapid plasma reagin) test was then one of the diagnostic criteria for lupus, of which I was blissfully ignorant.

As I noted, lupus is believed to result from a combination of genetic predisposition and an infectious trigger. The latter was possibly typhoid fever, which I contracted at age eleven during another family trip to India. I was hospitalized in D.C. for one month, as American doctors could not diagnose the cause of my fevers. My Indian-trained physician uncle flew in from abroad and promptly diagnosed this tropical infection. I received the appropriate antibiotic treatment and quickly recovered.

Meanwhile, my immune system had been overstimulated for close to two months. In attempting to fight the infection, autoantibodies were generated. Soon after, at age twelve, I was diagnosed with my first autoimmune condition, Hashimoto's thyroiditis. Interestingly, my only paternal aunt with a more limited form of lupus had also suffered a bad case of typhoid in childhood.

My psychiatry textbook hypothesized that autoimmune diseases such as rheumatoid arthritis or lupus may result from "suppressed rage." This blaming of the victim and the "pop science" notion that autoimmune disease is triggered mainly by psychological issues makes no sense. It ignores the fact that many people experience neglect, abuse, or other ordeals in childhood, but the vast majority do not develop autoimmune diseases. Yet again, we lupus warriors should NOT blame ourselves!

* * *

During my fourth year of medical school, which mainly entailed rotations that did not require overnight hospital duty, my symptoms improved markedly. This reassured me that I could handle internal medicine residency and that the condition might be remitting. My rheumatologist fully supported me in pursuing internal medicine, as there was no significant organ disease at that point.

The internship, which is the first year of residency, was far more physically, mentally, and emotionally challenging than medical school. On-call nights ranged from every second night to mostly every fourth night spent in the hospital, and we interns were at the hospital over eighty to one hundred hours a week. My symptoms worsened from the decreased ability to rest. By around 11:00 p.m. on call, I often developed painful inflammation of the joints of my ankles and feet. I had occasional red petechial rashes on the lower legs due to bleeding into the skin from the rupture of tiny, inflamed blood vessels. Snatching even a few hours of rest alleviated my symptoms significantly, and I was usually able to manage this.

During that era, even more than now, physicians were expected to be indefatigable. There was little compassion from the establishment towards underlings. The attitude was that we had to suffer just as they had and that our needs were secondary to those of our patients. Having adapted to this mindset as a medical student, I painfully overworked myself.

I continued to ignore my illness, though I saw my rheumatologist every three months for the necessary laboratory monitoring. I did not share my struggle with many of my fellow residents and friends. I feared being perceived as inadequate, accepting the unhealthy belief inculcated in medical school that we had to be strong, heroic, perfect, and self-sacrificing. No accommodation could have been made then, and I didn't want to burden my fellow residents with extra work because of my illness.

Surprisingly, none of my supervising attending physicians ever bothered to ask if I was all right, partly due to my success in concealing my illness. Three of my male fellow interns left internal medicine for careers in radiology at the end of their internship, finding the rigorous schedule and patient care far too stressful. Based on my own and fellow residents' experiences, I was determined to treat my trainees as humanely as possible. We physicians sometimes lack empathy for ourselves and each other—a culture crying out for reform.

The only time I ever missed work during my residency was during a month of emergency room duty when we alternated twelve-hour daytime shifts for six days one week with twelve hours of night duty the following week. One night, I awakened with a red, hot, swollen wrist, which was extremely painful and made it impossible for me to function. I was forced to call in sick, as I couldn't work. My poor friend and colleague that I was supposed to relieve ended up remaining at the hospital several hours past her shift until the "relief" resident appeared.

Concerned by the occasional severity of my fatigue and joint symptoms and though I loved my work, I asked my rheumatologist whether she would recommend a change of specialty to protect my health. Sleep deprivation and long work hours were taking a toll, and I was concerned that permanent injury might result. By then, I had also developed secondary Sjogren's syndrome, an autoimmune condition that often accompanies lupus. It primarily causes dry eyes and mouth due to autoimmune destruction of the lacrimal (tear) and salivary glands.

My rheumatologist reassured me that though my labs were markedly abnormal and indicated a high degree of inflammation, my lupus case was mild. I had primarily arthritis (joint inflammation) and rashes, with no involvement of the most common organ affected, the kidneys. Her assessment was that the pattern of lupus was "set in the first few years of the disease." She believed that since I was close to the end of the most grueling year of training with no kidney involvement, there was no need to switch specialties unless I was unhappy with internal medicine. I trained at an excellent east coast hospital with one of the country's top-rated rheumatology centers, demonstrating that the devious wolf can fool even the experts.

Fortunately, the years of training following the internship (i.e., residency) offered a respite. About half of the year was spent on hospital duty and the other half on consultative services, requiring only daytime hours. I was usually able to arrange my schedule to alternate the difficult and easier months, allowing for needed recovery. Fortunately, soon after I completed training, the training model altered, as residents unionized to demand more humane treatment—an overdue change.

Medicine is an arduous and humbling profession and may not be the best choice for one who has an illness aggravated by stress. Physicians tend to be self-critical and occasionally second-guess themselves when our patients do poorly, even when we're not at fault. I was guilty of this, too, as well as sometimes being overly involved emotionally. I am incredibly grateful that I survived the strenuous training years despite my inability to care for myself ideally. I now know of two lupus warriors who were not as fortunate, dying during their medical training.

The strain of a medical career likely accounts for the high suicide rate for physicians, especially women, compared to the general population. In the U.S., physicians are the profession with the highest suicide rate, with roughly 400 suicides yearly. High rates of alcohol and drug use are also a problem. Witnessing suffering, feeling impotent to help in many cases, and lack of self-compassion are all factors. Fear of litigation and concern that seeking mental health treatment may affect licensure also play a role. Physicians' stoic, perfectionist culture of disregarding our challenges aggravates the situation.

* * *

I am fortunate to have a very supportive and caring family. My mother and brother were sometimes frantic with worry over my decision to continue in a rigorous training program. At one point, my loving and concerned sibling said he feared losing me. He asked me to consider switching to a less demanding specialty or changing careers. My parents occasionally drove four hours from D.C. to Pittsburgh to visit and bring me food.

My mother, a warm, nurturing, typical Indian homemaker, has obsessed her entire life with the adequacy of my food intake—even now! Whenever visiting, she made and froze an ample supply of delicious food. During a very difficult period of persistent joint swelling and fatigue, Amma (Mom) came and spent a week helping me, enabling me to work and return home to sleep and recover.

My father dealt with my illness by never discussing it and looking sad whenever the subject arose. Though he was generally supportive and willing to help when I needed it, he had a strange relationship with illness. A proud man, he had no patience with weakness of any kind. Appa (Dad) didn't truly understand lupus due to its invisibility, which was painful for me.

For example, when I visited my parents on vacation, I would sleep as late as 9:00 a.m. some mornings due to exhaustion. Amma conveyed that Appa thought this was unacceptable and considered me undisciplined. He believed that with sufficient motivation, one could overcome any challenge, just as he had conquered many obstacles in his life.

Relationships can be fraught for all of us and require a considerable time investment. With lupus and other chronic debilitating illnesses, the challenges multiply. A good relationship is certainly worth the effort, but my condition contributed to some poor decisions, which didn't serve me well. Instead, they increased the tensions in my life, which we lupus warriors know can aggravate the disease. The culture clash imposed by my family further complicated my relationship choices.

My brother had recently married a fantastic American, and my father refused to attend the ceremony because she was not Hindu. My father also forbid my mother from going, though I and extended family and friends attended. I knew then that though I didn't wish to be restricted by my father's religious inflexibility, it was unsettling to imagine marrying without my parents' presence.

It was unclear whether my father would ever accept my sister-in-law, and my mother was distraught at the prospect of losing both her children. Fortunately, a few years later, when my nephew was born, all was forgiven by my father. Had I known this reconciliation would occur, I may have made different choices from the ones I will soon relate.

I had an amazing, idealistic boyfriend in medical school who grew up in public housing and won a scholarship to a top east coast university. It was my first serious relationship, and we talked about marriage. Sadly, we broke up after the internship for several reasons.

As a budding surgeon, he believed that his career was more important than mine and that my dreams were secondary to his. He expected that we would relocate as needed to advance his career. As I wanted a partnership of equals, this was a problem. He also made it clear that he would never forgive my parents for failing to accept him initially. Though we loved each other, I realized the relationship was unworkable.

My parents were relieved about the breakup, but I then faced intense pressure from them to marry. By then, it seemed far less complicated to marry someone everyone would be happy about rather than fracture our family. Furthermore, lupus made me feel vulnerable, as its disabling symptoms could make single life very difficult. I feared being alone, though unwilling to admit this to myself. As Indian parents often do, they had unpleasantly "surprised" me during my brief visits home by introducing me to a few young Hindu Indian men.

One of these men made an impression on me, as he seemed kind, charming, and engaging, and we developed a connection. Although I was on the rebound, I contacted him soon after ending the other relationship, knowing he lived nearby. As with all my relationships, I was open with him regarding lupus, my symptoms, and its potential to worsen. We dated for about a year, engaged, and married before I completed my residency. I later realized that married life also carries many stressors and complexities, sometimes more than single life.

One dilemma I contended with was that lupus and my health status might affect my ability to obtain employment—a challenge we warriors often face. As a senior resident, I began getting phone calls from headhunters in Ohio. We planned to move there as my husband, with more limited options as an engineer, secured an ideal job there. One recruiter asked if I was in good health, and as I had completed a rigorous training program, I hesitated but responded affirmatively.

Due to my hesitation, the headhunters called my department chairman with questions about my health. My boss met with me to tell me that my health status was my business and that I shouldn't discuss it with any prospective employer. I had missed only one twelve-hour shift during my three-year residency, and he knew I was a reliable, knowledgeable, and capable physician respected by my peers and supervisors.

A few months before completing training, I noticed that my urinalysis lab report showed blood, which my doctor hadn't mentioned. Using a centrifuge, I spun down my urine and analyzed the cellular sediment with a microscope. I was alarmed to see red blood cell casts indicating I had glomerulonephritis, a severe kidney complication of lupus. I wondered if I was facing eventual kidney failure and resulting disability. I had cared for many patients requiring hemodialysis and couldn't imagine dependency on an artificial kidney for about twelve hours a week.

Though frightened, I knew that most dialysis patients eventually feel they have a reasonable quality of life, as we humans are amazingly resilient. Studies in patients with spinal cord injury resulting in paralysis, for example, find that people typically experience a year-long grieving period. After this, they return to their baseline level of contentment.

Similar studies have been done with HIV patients before treatments were developed, rendering it a chronic illness. These patients reported that their concept of a tolerable quality of life also changed over time. They no longer wanted the "do not resuscitate" status they selected earlier in their illness. Their survival instinct overcame concerns about living with a disability. "Hedonic adaptation" is the term psychologists use for this altered perspective.

I underwent a kidney biopsy to evaluate the urine abnormalities, and it showed some scarring in the kidney due to lupus glomerulonephritis with no ongoing injury. Given this flare and exhaustion from residency, I opted to take a few months off between training and starting a job. I then began intensely missing work and saw an ad for a local urgent care center that offered flexible hours. I started working there three to four days weekly, doing eight-to-nine-hour shifts, with some spacing between shifts to prevent exhaustion. Gradually, I began exercising regularly to optimize my fitness.

Unfortunately, my kidney function continued to deteriorate over the next six months, and I was treated with high-dose steroids for several months. I developed pneumonia due to the steroids and was forced to take medical leave from the job I had just started. I was very discouraged, fearing my hard work, training, and enthusiasm for medicine were for nothing. My nephrologist (kidney specialist) kindly tried to encourage me, but given the unpredictability of lupus, there was nothing he could say that was very reassuring.

To further evaluate my pneumonia, I underwent a bronchoscopy procedure to look for unusual or "opportunistic" infections, which can occur in patients on immunosuppressing drugs such as steroids. These organisms typically don't cause infection in those with a healthy immune system. Fortunately, nothing unusual turned up, and the condition was resolved with antibiotics.

After the infection had resolved, I returned to the urgent care job. I enjoyed the work but missed having ongoing relationships with patients. After a year, I learned of an opportunity to join the internal medicine faculty at the local medical school, the University of Cincinnati College of Medicine. This job would entail caring for patients both in and outside the hospital and teaching medical students and residents. As it's a large public hospital, the patient population is diverse socioeconomically and racially, which met my goals. I discovered a love of teaching during my training, as everyone on the medical team taught the less experienced.

Throughout this period, I was intermittently anxious about end-stage kidney failure, which would require dialysis or a transplant. My husband, mother, and brother generously offered to donate a kidney to me if needed, as their blood types are compatible with mine. Eventually, the kidney function stabilized at an abnormal but adequate level, to my great relief. Soon after, I developed hypertension (high blood pressure) secondary to my kidney disease.

The inspiring courage of many patients helped me cope with kidney disease. I'd seen patients younger than me deal with far more dire situations with immense bravery. One of many examples is a twenty-year-old with acute leukemia (blood cancer), who often required evaluation by me for high fevers in the middle of the night. On one occasion, my exhaustion was evident to him, and the following day he shared that he felt concerned that I worked so hard—remarkable selflessness from someone so ill.

A few days later, my patient suddenly stopped breathing, requiring a ventilator and intensive care unit transfer. I sobbed at the nurses' station while the older attending oncologist sadly watched me. Especially in those days, cancer patients had very little chance of surviving critical illness, though currently, outcomes have improved.

In moments of self-pity, which most of us with chronic illness experience, I recall the images and words of many who have amazed me with their extraordinary affirmation of life while facing illness. I've treated people of all races and ethnicities and have observed that my older Black women patients are especially remarkable in their ability to remain grateful, regardless of their hardships. Even those with little resources, serious illness, and family problems invariably responded, "I'm blessed!" when replying to my query about how they felt.

This first renal (kidney) injury reinforced the most valuable rule in coping with lupus: the importance of listening to my body and getting the rest it demands rather than abusing it to serve my mind. Taking care of others has always felt healing, as it does for most of us, but it can't be at our own expense. Perhaps for some of us, it's easier to help others than to analyze and attend to our needs. A friend shared the Jewish saying, "If I am not for myself, who will be for me?" to make the point that I first had to take care of myself. This is a lesson that has been sometimes forgotten in my decades of living with the wolf.

A Dream Fulfilled

"The primary work of a professor of medicine in a medical school is in the wards, teaching his pupils how to deal with patients and their diseases."

— Sir William Osler

My initial position at the U.C. College of Medicine was at the rehabilitation, extended acute care, and long-term care hospital affiliated with the university. It involved providing medical consultation to U.C. staff physical medicine and rehabilitation physicians, caring for ill, ventilator-dependent patients, and nursing home residents. Realizing my early unhealthy denial of my diagnosis didn't serve me well, I learned to be open with coworkers and friends and solicit the support I needed. Allowing pride to interfere with self-care is a losing and risky strategy, so I shared my challenge with colleagues in case of significant flares.

I saw this opportunity as an ideal way to get my foot in the door of the local university medical center with a reasonable, manageable schedule. Internal medicine residents rotated at the hospital so that I could teach again, and I also led trainees on hospital rounds one month a year at the university hospital. Though I took night calls every four to five nights, an onsite doctor was first called after hours, with only occasional calls coming to the staff doctors.

Initially, the variety of patients was interesting. I especially enjoyed the challenge of helping chronically ventilator-reliant patients wean from their dependency. There were tragic cases of young people suffering severe traumatic brain injuries, some from driving drunk. On the other extreme were elderly patients who had suffered catastrophic events such as massive strokes.

Some patients adapted incredibly well to their drastically altered conditions. For example, a kind, older man had fallen from his roof, resulting in quadriplegia. He was completely paralyzed and unable to breathe independently. He possessed a tranquil spirit and calmly accepted his severe disability, smiling at everyone he saw. Aiding in his adjustment to his new circumstances, he soon began working on his memoirs with the help of a relative.

We celebrated discharges to home, which occurred infrequently. After I'd been there a few years, yet another young man was admitted in a vegetative state from a traumatic brain injury. Upon entering the room and seeing the bedside photo of him with his young wife and baby, I broke down in tears. At this point, I realized it was time for me to leave and resume outpatient medical practice. I was experiencing burnout and could not continue to cope effectively with the steady stream of depressing, disastrous, and heartbreaking tragedies I was seeing.

During these years, my husband (now my ex-husband) and I decided to start a family. We considered our options, as my lupus had been stable long enough to become a mother. As I love children, my goal was to be a parent, rather than to propagate my genes. Moreover, pregnancy with lupus kidney disease carries some health risks. In India, as in some other countries, girls are considered a burden upon their families and abandoned more often than boys. Weighing these factors, we decided to adopt a baby girl from India.

At this point, my husband expressed uncertainty about whether he was too selfish to be a parent, though he'd firmly committed to the notion before we married. He seemed simply nervous about the significant life change. After discussion and some gentle persuasion on my part, he agreed to proceed and seemed genuinely excited.

The bureaucracy in India was unbelievably inefficient and delayed the adoption process, causing me heartache. I grieved daily, thinking of my baby alone in the children's home. Although we had agreed to adopt the newborn within a day of her entry there, Maya finally arrived home to us at thirteen months of age. Adapting quickly, Maya was sleeping through the night by then, the one consolation in her late arrival. With lupus, the sleep deprivation involved in awakening to feed an infant could have been problematic.

Welcoming her was and still is the happiest event of my life. Five years earlier, with my first kidney flare, I felt uncertain about my future health, and parenthood. Now, my already beloved daughter was with me! Parenting has been my single greatest challenge and one of my life's most significant sources of purpose. They warned us at the children's home that Maya would be a handful. By nine months of age, when the other infants were sleeping, she was striding around the place, acting like she was in command!

Maya had many disruptions in her young life including separation from her birth mother, living in the children's home, and then traveling half a world away to her new family. Her temperament quickly became apparent, and she was loving and engaging, rapidly bonding with us. She was also astonishingly strong-willed. One morning, within her first few weeks at home, she decided she didn't want to get dressed. She flailed about angrily, refusing to cooperate and forcing me to wait a few hours until she was in a better mood. Much to my consternation, Maya established early on that she was in charge!

As she grew, she was oppositional, refusing to go into time out when she misbehaved. I hoped this would bode well for her future and that she would never allow anyone to mistreat her, but it made for some rough parental challenges. She was prone to frequent tantrums and histrionics, which I coped with by remaining calm and trying to soothe her. There was also love, joy, and laughter amidst the trials.

Maya showed an extraordinary love of animals from a very young age. Raised by two dog-phobic parents, I was determined not to model this fear to my child. She bonded with neighborhood dogs from infancy and began volunteering at our local animal shelter by age nine. Naturally, she fell in love with the dogs and wanted to bring them home. Over time I overcame my apprehension and learned to love them too. Dogs have been an essential part of our households ever since.

As a child, my daughter was sometimes understandably annoyed that I lacked the energy to do everything she wanted. I shared that I had lupus, which limited my energy—difficult for an active child to grasp. Our families sometimes want to pursue pastimes so much that they urge us to do what's not feasible. I occasionally find this even now in my household. It's tough for those who love us to process and accept our limitations.

I hadn't shared much about the disease's potential complications with Maya, as we don't want to burden our children. She knew I was more fatigued and required naps and rest more than her friends' moms. Looking back, explaining the illness more to her over time may have been wiser than trying to protect her. We warriors must find the elusive balance between being participating family members and risking our health by overdoing it. The disappointment we feel over our constraints also calls for tremendous patience with ourselves.

As an adult, my daughter had a young coworker, newly diagnosed with lupus, whose husband didn't understand the disease. She looked fine to him, so why did she claim she didn't feel well? Soon after, the young woman quit, unable to continue working. Maya then gained a greater comprehension of lupus and apologized for being difficult at times in childhood. She has matured into a beautiful, loving, joyful, and responsible young adult.

Educating your loved ones, especially household members, about lupus is essential. Sharing your symptoms and what's at risk fosters their understanding, cooperation, and assistance. It also helps reduce resentment over your inability to consistently carry your share of household duties.

Resist the tendency many of us have to downplay our condition to avoid worrying or burdening others. This doesn't serve us well, as we need family support. Conversely, we don't need to complain constantly though we may rarely feel well! It can be more complicated for women warriors, who usually carry a greater share of the household load than our partners.

We patients are all used to being told we look fine and healthy, as we may have chubby cheeks from steroid use. Most people are unfamiliar with lupus, but those who have heard of it generally believe it just causes fatigue. Friends, neighbors, and acquaintances sometimes wonder aloud why we're not working or only working part-time, though close friends are more sensitive.

We're all accustomed to hearing things like, "Why don't you just exercise more. That would give you more energy," and "How can you sleep so much?" or "Well, you can't be that bad, since you're not bedridden." Upon hearing these questions and well-meaning advice, I'm reminded of how it felt to get parenting guidance from childless friends. Certainly, lupus can be about as tamable as a two-year-old amid a tantrum!

Funny misunderstandings can also occur, such as when a friend and I took our girls to summer camp two hours away. I fell asleep about a half hour into the trip and was mortified to awaken only when we arrived. I apologized, explaining that I had lupus. She completely understood and chuckled, saying she had assumed she was just a boring conversationalist!

* * *

After a brief transition period, I was thrilled and honored to join the premier faculty practice at the university. The only potential problem this presented was that my workload would increase. I would have to take night calls every fifth night and weekend, which my partners assured me was a light task with an average of three calls per weeknight and perhaps fifteen per weekend. Resuming outpatient practice was everything I had hoped in choosing internal medicine, with the combination of long-term relationships with patients and intellectual stimulation.

In patient care, prevention of illness is one of my priorities. We served both indigent and insured patients in our practice, and I had many patients with severe chronic illnesses. We also received referrals from community doctors of patients with illnesses that were difficult to diagnose or treat. Over time, the number of underserved patients grew as the "concierge" or "boutique" medical practice model became more popular in Cincinnati.

This model caused us to be increasingly inundated with desperate patients who could not afford the monthly retainer fees newly required by their physicians. My group and I believe physicians have an ethical responsibility to care for all people of diverse backgrounds and means. The national increase of the concierge practice tremendously strains conventional doctors, leaving many patients struggling to access care.

I managed my new schedule, though I was chronically mildly fatigued and had occasional joint pain, muscle pain, and infrequent joint swelling. I managed to get ten hours of sleep nightly, plus afternoon naps on weekends. As I was young, determined, and lucky, I pushed through.

Taking night calls made uninterrupted sleep a challenge, as there were usually some in the middle of the night. Fortunately, I was able to wake quickly, respond to the problem, and promptly fall back asleep—the result of years of training as a resident and the advantage of youth. Interestingly, some rheumatologists have noted that the onset of kidney disease makes the overall symptoms of lupus less severe, which I experienced.

However, my symptoms continued, and there were times I had the flu-like "malaise" that lupus patients know well. Like severe fatigue, malaise causes you to " hit a wall" and be forced to lie down and sleep. Rarely, I had to get to bed right after dinner, requiring a solid twelve-to-thirteen-hour rest for the night. Chest pains associated with deep breathing or coughing (pleuritic pain) occurred transiently and infrequently.

Due to secondary Sjogren's syndrome, I had chronic (long-standing) eye redness, irritation, and pain. To clarify, Sjogren's syndrome can occur on its own, but when it occurs along with lupus, it is referred to as secondary Sjogren's. Episcleritis, an autoimmune inflammation of the layer below the superficial layer of the eye, aggravated the redness. I began developing frequent bouts of conjunctivitis at one point and required preventive bedtime ocular (eye) antibiotics for several years. Dry mouth, also from Sjogren's, led to many cavities and the need for crowns over the decades, despite excellent self-care.

My lung problems also gradually worsened, with bronchiectasis, a form of COPD, developing in addition to the mild interstitial lung disease. As a general internist, I was exposed to many patients with respiratory infections and developed frequent infections myself. Wearing masks was not routine in those days, though my office introduced them over time for the infectious patient. Due to my lung disease, most of my colds led to a secondary bacterial infection, and I had recurrent bronchitis and rarely, pneumonia.

These infections caused further lung scarring, and I developed mild shortness of breath with exertion. I suffered a few attacks of hemoptysis (coughing up blood) over these decades, associated with brief episodes of shortness of breath and chest pain. These necessitated CT (computerized tomography) scans to rule out lung blood clots, as lupus can increase that risk. Though I have some antibodies predisposing me to blood clots, fortunately, I have not had this complication.

My pulmonologist placed me on a preventive daily dose of antibiotics, which reduced my bouts of viral infection by diminishing the bacterial load and inflammation in my lungs. Later, after getting much sicker and becoming unable to work full-time, I no longer required this preventive treatment. Eliminating the high degree of exposure to infection was clearly beneficial.

Practicing medicine at the university was deeply rewarding, and it was a tremendous privilege to be entrusted with people's most personal problems and struggles. Over time, I cared for multiple family members and several generations. Like other healthcare professionals, I sometimes had difficulty maintaining detachment from my patients and the many tragedies I witnessed. At graduation, the dean of my medical school reminded us that the secret of exemplary patient care is genuinely caring for our patients, which thankfully comes easily to me.

I went to work mentally exhilarated but a little tired each day and returned home fatigued but fulfilled. Even when my daughter was relatively young, she commented on my love of work and the enjoyment it brought me. She contrasted this with a neighbor, whom she characterized as "grumpy," saying she wouldn't want to have him for a doctor.

Diagnostic dilemmas and assisting patients to control long-term conditions are gratifying. There is great purpose in helping people and working to alleviate suffering, as there are still many incurable diseases. Some patients said they considered me part of their family. This mutual affection was one of the treasured aspects of my work.

Despite the many rewards, medicine is a stressful profession. When advising my lupus patients regarding career choices, I suggest considering the flexibility to care for oneself. As you have seen, this is a lesson I was slow to internalize.

The other central aspect of my work was teaching medical students and residents in hospital and clinic settings. Sir

William Osler, considered the father of modern medicine, commented that he felt his most significant contribution was teaching. As reliance on testing has increased, more than ever, trainees need to learn good clinical skills. Listening to the patient is one of the most valuable diagnostic tools, and a thorough physical examination is also important. As students and trainees pored over test results, they occasionally needed a reminder to speak with and examine the patient carefully.

Also critical, I felt, was teaching my trainees by example to treat every patient with respect, dignity, and compassion. My illness helped me become a more empathetic physician, as I could relate to being on the receiving end of doctors' visits, hospitalizations, and procedures. In the increasingly technology-dependent world of medicine, our shared humanity is becoming a casualty. The healing power of listening, touching, and being present with our patients' suffering is immeasurable.

My teaching evaluations from medical students and doctors in training were excellent overall, and some said I was the best teacher in their medical careers. They included comments about how moved they were by my compassion and efforts to help our patients in any way possible. I had been fortunate to learn from some fantastic teachers in medical school and residency who served as role models.

U.C. is primarily an indigent care hospital, though it also has the reputation of being *the* place to go in Cincinnati if one were extremely ill or had a perplexing condition. We had a large share of the homeless and incarcerated patients in the city. Like many of my colleagues, I disliked the propensity of some doctors to cater to wealthy patients, giving them preferential treatment.

For example, during residency, a senior faculty physician came down to the E.R. and asked us to "roll out the red carpet" for his "VIP" patient who would soon arrive. We residents joked that we would roll out the red biohazard material trash bags, as we had no use for differential treatment of patients. Unfortunately, as in our society, bias, discrimination, and elitism are problems for all of us in medicine. The profession is working to confront these issues with the goal of more equitable care.

The Relentlessness of the Wolf

"We must be willing to let go of the life we have planned so that we can accept the one that is waiting for us."

— Joseph Campbell

I found that handling the physical challenges of lupus becomes more taxing with age. By my late forties, I required very low-dose steroids chronically in addition to Plaquenil (hydroxychloroquine), which I started in my late twenties. As time went on, I increasingly required accommodations at work with my hospital ward schedule.

I initially performed one month of ward attending, leading and teaching a team of up to eight or so medical students and trainee physicians. Hospital rounds occurred daily for the entire month, including weekends. At times, this could mean five straight weeks of working every single day. Fortunately, weekend rounds typically required only half a day.

My ward attending rotation was always a physically and psychologically trying month, as our outpatient responsibilities continued with a truncated schedule. This duty involved considerable walking, too, as patients could be on any hospital floor. This was possible in my early years on the faculty, though I was fatigued and in pain by the end of this month-long increase in workload and physical demands.

Progressively, as I aged, I began to flare with arthritis and exhaustion by the middle of the month's hospital duty, and I requested two two-week blocks instead, splitting the rotation with a colleague. Over time, this became the norm for most attending physicians, as it was far more workable. After all, many of us were over the age of forty or fifty, and working over sixty hours a week is difficult for many.

By my late forties, I reluctantly gave up ward attending work altogether, as I began to flare soon into my two-week block. This was very disappointing, as hospital work and the teaching involved are fascinating and fulfilling. Instead, I increased my outpatient teaching duties. Having physician colleagues who understood lupus symptoms helped me obtain these necessary changes over time, which, woefully, many patients cannot do.

* * *

It became clear over the years that my marriage was failing, as my husband chose less and less involvement with me or our daughter. He urged us to leave the house on weekends so that he could watch sports, read newspapers, and have time to himself. The rejection of living with someone who pays the family little attention was heart-wrenching. Children know when their parents are unhappy, and though there was never any yelling or abuse, the growing tension became more difficult for Maya.

Initially, I tried to share my needs with him, and he acknowledged them and improved his behavior for a few days. But he was incapable of sustaining it, and his lack of interest even extended to his birth family. He rarely, if ever, called his parents or siblings. I later learned that his family said, "No one knows him at all!"

He could be a charming person but quite a chameleon. When dating, he quickly gauged my priorities and claimed he shared my views. He was funny and engaging, and we seemed to have much in common. He talked about his love of children and desire to have a family. In the early years of our marriage, he seemed to be the person I fell in love with, but over time, it became more evident that he was highly self-absorbed.

Having my father as a standard of comparison, I rationalized that at least he wasn't unkind in his speech. In fact, though, he had very little to say to us! My father was a loving, engaged parent and husband, though temperamental. Over time, I realized how hurtful my husband's passive aggression was and that emotional intimacy was beyond him. He repeatedly told me he loved me, but his concept of a loving relationship bore no resemblance to mine. Still, I deluded myself that we could work through this together.

Our families sometimes don't fathom what we're experiencing as lupus patients. My husband sometimes implied I was a hypochondriac, saying I'd probably outlive everyone in the family. He was fearful of hospitals and spent all of two minutes with me when I was hospitalized for a kidney biopsy.

It takes integrity, empathy, and a generous spirit to remain happily partnered with a chronically ill person. I've seen situations in which sick women have been abandoned by their male partners. As most cultures assign females the nurturing caregiver role, this is unsurprising. These qualities exist in men, too, though they are not often socialized to develop them.

My marital unhappiness was apparent to my family during visits, and they asked me why I remained in the relationship. This was extraordinary coming from my mother, who, thirty years earlier, warned me against divorce! I responded that raising a young child alone as a lupus patient was a daunting prospect. I suspect my ex-husband believed that my disease trapped me. Gradually, I desensitized myself to my feelings about the marriage and grew increasingly numb as I focused on work and raising Maya.

Finally, when Maya was eight, I acknowledged there was no hope of salvaging the relationship. The efforts were one-sided, and he was too "busy" with work to seek counseling for his mild depression or to continue couples counseling after only two sessions. He constantly undermined the reasonable limits I placed on Maya, confusing her.

Shortly before the separation was official, he was away on business for a week. Upon his return, Maya said, "Daddy, go away. Mom's a lot happier when you're not here!" I asked him to move out, which I'd been considering for a few months. Obviously, the situation was detrimental to my mental and potentially physical health and Maya's well-being.

He was incredulous that I believed I could manage Maya and the household independently, as he helped with chores. To my surprise, he said our years together were the happiest of his life, and he wanted to save our marriage. He then said he would fully participate in counseling after repeatedly abandoning and refusing it. His intentions were good, but he could not carry them out. It was too little too late. We agreed that I would have custody of Maya, and he would have visitation rights every other weekend and one weeknight.

Divorce is always far more stressful than anticipated, and mine was no exception. Concern about being alone for the rest of my life played a role in my grief, as I was only forty-two years old. My dream of the happy family life lacking in my childhood was shattered. Naively, I had believed that the high divorce rate in our country resulted from a lack of motivation to make a marriage work. In some partnerships, basic incompatibility cannot be overcome, especially with a one-sided effort.

As emotional and physical exhaustion lead to lupus flares, I was fortunate not to have a severe flare around the time of my divorce. There was undoubtedly stress relief as well, as it's painful to have someone present in your home who is withdrawn from the family. This was a reminder that the more chronically ill can be extra vulnerable in relationships. It's essential to guard against victimization by partners who believe we will tolerate their neglect or abuse. The stakes are higher for us lupus warriors since divorce is one of life's major stressors.

Over my years in practice, I've seen patients whose partners abused them physically and emotionally. A wheelchair-bound older woman had an abusive, alcoholic husband but concealed it from me. When she came in with a black eye, it was clear what was happening, but she continued to ignore it, claiming she "ran into her furniture."

All I could do was urge her to deal with it, as it would surely escalate, and provide her with resources for help. Finally, several months later, she sought aid and left the marriage to move in with her daughter and her family. Unsurprisingly, she shared that her disability had made divorce more frightening and financially prohibitive.

This was one of many situations in which my female patients dealt with abuse. Another patient shared that my divorce inspired her to leave her emotionally abusive husband, deciding she could do it if I did! As I returned to my maiden name, my patients knew I had divorced. They began to share more of their relationship difficulties, which in some cases impacted their mental and physical health.

* * *

Knowing Amma needed ongoing support, I checked in with her briefly each day. Throughout my career, she kept reminding me to take care of myself and often suggested working part-time, especially when I sounded more tired than usual. Though Amma was trying to be helpful, I did what we sometimes do in these situations—I simply let her do all the worrying for me. Meanwhile, my indoctrination as a physician had already taught me to minimize my needs.

After my divorce, I began exploring dating options as I was still young and knew that a mutually loving relationship was possible. One of my friends said she wouldn't even bother, but I value companionship. I learned about the online dating service eHarmony and that it successfully brought compatible people together. It is based on the research of Ph.D. psychologists with vast experience in marital counseling, and I knew of a few physicians who were happily married as a result.

After two years, I'd had no success and began reconciling myself to a reasonably contented single life. I then met a wonderful person, Dan. His fascinating profile showed we had much in common: we were both vegetarians, had similar political views, a love of nature, enjoyed learning and reading, and shared a sense of humor. We knew early on that we had an extraordinary connection.

After our first few months together, Dan mentioned he had been researching lupus to understand the disease better and how it affected me. He also offered to donate one of his kidneys to me immediately! Laughing, I told him I didn't need it yet, but I appreciated the kind offer. We are still happily together more than fifteen years later, and he is amazingly giving, remaining by my side through my life-threatening flare and beyond. He's been steadfast even through complications posing a threat of severe disability or worse, as I'll describe later.

As often happens, Maya was resistant to the presence of another person in our lives. She had no use for another parental figure who might distract me from her, though she also complained that I gave her too much attention! However, she was perceptive and understood that I would enjoy adult companionship. A friend who was a professor of developmental psychology assured me that it takes about ten years for blended families to come together, so I simply had to be patient. Sure enough, that's just how long it took.

* * *

The advent of EMR, or electronic medical records, was heralded as an advance that would improve patient care by sharing patient records. It was also supposed to lead to tremendous cost savings in healthcare by eliminating the replication of testing and services. When my medical center rolled this out in 2006, it was a simple, doctors' office-based system that was very user-friendly and to which we readily adapted. It was a different story in 2012 when an extensive system covering hospitals and clinics was instituted.

As the new system was being introduced nationally in many centers, there was a dearth of training staff, and we physicians were left to train ourselves. EMR was designed by computer engineers with no meaningful input from physicians. The primary focus of the system seemed to be to ensure billing was completely "captured" to maximize profits for the institution. It shifted the clerical work of ordering tests from nurses and medical assistants to doctors—not the best utilization of our time and skill set.

There were many glitches that neither the supplier nor most institutions were equipped to deal with, leaving doctors struggling. Some older doctors who were unaccustomed to computers found it insurmountable, with burnout and early retirement increasing. For example, one of the worst problems was that even after checking boxes to indicate that lab tests and studies had been examined, they continually reappeared on the screen, requiring repeated review. It felt like we were in our own irritating version of *Groundhog Day*. For those familiar, in this comedy, the same day unfolds each time the actors awaken.

EMR quickly added hours to our daily schedules, as studies have confirmed. Face-to-face connections have been strained, leaving physicians and patients alike dissatisfied. One study found that for every hour spent with patients, outpatient physicians spend nearly two hours performing EMR documentation and paperwork. This is in addition to one to two hours nightly spent on administrative work.[4] Our digital society has indeed taken over every realm we inhabit, even those where a trusting, empathetic relationship can be healing. The depersonalization of physicians' focus on a computer may also discourage patients from discussing sensitive, critical issues that should be addressed. These include, for example, sexual, psychological, or domestic abuse problems.

It's no exaggeration to say that using electronic medical records played a role in my first major, life-threatening flare of 2013. EMR had been in place for eight months, and I, along with my partners in practice, had grown increasingly tired and overwhelmed. Some occasionally fell asleep around midnight, computers in our laps, trying to complete medical record charting at home. More lucrative sub-specialty doctors hired scribes to do all their documentation, making their lives far more manageable. Like many female doctors, I maintained eye contact with patients. Maintaining rapport with my patients is important but added to my work hours.

My "elite" academic practice was predominantly male and white. It included the head of the department of internal medicine, a dean of the medical school, and the leading physician in the hospital administration. I was the first minority female in the group, and as we minority women well know, we must be tough and more than capable of proving our worth. I had no interest in the political maneuverings in the department or trying to move up the hierarchy, as patient care and teaching have always been my passion. However, I was always conscious of the need to do my part to contribute to the group effort to care for our patients.

I had my regular three-month visit with my lupus doctor in December of that year. I mentioned that I was more fatigued than usual. He asked if I felt I needed a short medical leave, which I didn't believe was necessary. I had previously had episodes of increased fatigue that improved while continuing to work. Since I didn't have my usual flare symptoms, including joint pain or swelling, I rationalized that there was nothing serious afoot.

My lab results showed no evidence of a flare, and my conscience wouldn't allow me to abandon my patients and partners. My colleagues were already terribly overworked and I feared would struggle to care for my patients. I was concerned and believed my fatigue did not justify increasing their workload. Everyone felt overburdened, with the strain evident on their faces.

Other stressors were unfolding simultaneously. Dan, who is ten years older than I, had planned for many years to move to California after retirement. He had already sold his small business but was willing to wait until Maya graduated from high school. As we were engaged by then, I agreed to move to California with Dan after Maya completed school.

Over the six months or so before the flare, I realized that continuing my work hours was becoming harder. By then, I was fifty years old and had found that age plus lupus made full-time work challenging. I planned to move, take a few months off, and resume working part-time.

Dan was fearful I wouldn't want to leave, knowing my love of my job and commitment to it and Maya. Knowing that I would need to give my colleagues ample notice, he began urging me to let my colleagues know I'd be departing in about a year and a half. So, I was in the midst of a perfect storm of physical and psychological stressors—a situation in which we warriors must be wary and deescalate tensions in any possible healthy way.

I was confident that Maya would be fine with my move, as she'd always been highly independent and generally rejected adult guidance. Telling my partners in January 2013 that I would leave in about eighteen months was one of the most stressful things I've had to do, as I had a great deal of loyalty to my patients and coworkers. One of my sisters-in-law reminded me that I had to "first put on my oxygen mask before helping others" and finally concentrate on *my* health.

The Wolf Pounces

"Nothing can happen to you that is not positive. Even though it looks and feels like a negative crisis at the moment, it is not. The crisis throws you back, and when you are required to exhibit strength, it comes."

– Joseph Campbell

Roughly two months after my rheumatologist visit and labs, I became sick at work. I developed chills, fever, and cough and went home with treatment from one of my doctors for a respiratory infection. The cough was improving, but I gradually worsened the following week. Over the weekend, I began passing pink urine, indicating the presence of blood. I also developed more shortness of breath than usual, which occasionally accompanied my respiratory infections but could have many other causes, including lupus flares.

In speaking with a dear friend and fellow internist from medical school, who is also a lupus warrior, I related that I needed to see my doctors due to worsening illness. She soon recognized how weak I sounded and was concerned about the blood in my urine. She insisted on flying in from 500 miles away the following morning. She accompanied me to my lupus doctor and nephrologist appointments along with Dan, who had just returned from California the night before.

Despite feeling poorly, I was confident of soon returning to work. The overwhelming fatigue with the flare was undoubtedly a factor in my lack of mental clarity, as well as brain fog. Brain fog is a slowing of thought processes and difficulty focusing that can accompany lupus flares and chronic lupus. Fortunately, it is not progressive and improves as flares subside. About 80 to 90 percent of lupus patients experience cognitive problems at some point.

My labs were rechecked and showed I was in rapidly progressive kidney failure. My immune system was also destroying my red blood cells, an unusual lupus complication referred to as autoimmune hemolytic anemia (AIHA). A recent study showed that kidney, blood, and multi-organ disease are more common in Asian and Latino lupus patients, though they can occur in anyone.[5]

A kidney biopsy was done very quickly, revealing crescentic glomerulonephritis, the most severe and aggressive form of lupus kidney disease. I began chemotherapy over the next three months. I also received blood transfusions because of anemia (low hemoglobin or red blood count), which was mainly due to the autoimmune destruction of my blood cells. The kidney failure, fortunately, responded well to the treatment, but the hemolytic anemia persisted. This necessitated the use of high-dose steroids for nearly six months and the initiation of mycophenolate, a potent immunosuppressant that treats lupus kidney disease and hemolytic anemia.

Here's Dan's reaction to my treatment:

"The chemotherapy treatment room looked like a hair salon but seeing Niranjana reclined there with her outstretched arm hooked to an I.V. (intravenous line) clearly defined the difference. Knowing that the I.V. bag was dripping cell-destroying chemicals into her frail body required some deep breathing, and convincing myself this was essential to keeping her alive.

This image was still clear as a few weeks later, we returned to the hospital for a similar picture. This time it was for blood transfusions. As I stood beside her with her small hand in mine and watched the IV bag empty, only to be followed by another, I felt guilty for my good health. I was furious that someone who dedicated her life to helping others had this incurable disease and was also anxious that I may not be capable of being the life partner she needed and deserved. I felt angry that this wolf-like disease was tearing apart the woman I loved."

During the first few months of this illness, I was sleeping about twenty hours a day and was so weak that my voice was a barely audible squeak. The combination of kidney failure and high-dose steroids, which cause the body to retain sodium and water, caused generalized swelling of my whole body. I joked that I looked like the Michelin woman.

My shortness of breath worsened for some time due to the inflammation from the flare, low blood count, and lung disease. Over time, my immune system also began destroying a subtype of my white blood cells, the lymphocytes. This has continued to wax and wane over the years, varying with the dose of immunosuppressants.

I showed slight improvement in my symptoms for several months. Due to my multi-organ complications, I saw a rheumatologist, nephrologist, hematologist (blood doctor), pulmonologist, and both general and cornea specialist ophthalmologists. Dan worried that I would never recover any strength, repeatedly asking if this might be my new baseline condition. It has been tough for Dan to accept that there's no cure for lupus. Maya was also worried but hid her concerns, repeatedly insisting that I would be "fine." My sweet dog Elsie lay by my side throughout my recovery, looking depressed by my illness. It helped that some kind friends brought us food and support.

Dan still likes to tell an amusing story about the ravenous, high-dose, steroid-induced appetite I experienced for several months. Knowing my fondness for pecan pie, some friends brought me one. I should have known better, but the steroids overcame my good sense. They watched in astonishment as I rapidly devoured more than a third of the pie! This is an excellent example of what *not* to do on steroids.

Sadly, my concern about being ill was almost outweighed by my fears of letting my patients and partners down. I obsessed over this. Although I knew I was very sick, I felt hopeful I'd recover with the combination of chemotherapy and immunosuppressants. Medicine has been a "calling" for me, making it almost my whole identity, and thus fearful of losing it.

My conscientiousness and pride had dire consequences, which eventually taught me much about myself and what to do differently in the future. The progression of my fatigue was so gradual and insidious that I had adapted to it. My twenty-two-year period of mild disease had allowed the sneaky wolf to fool me into complacency—something for all of us to guard against.

The "able-bodied" individual is widely considered more valuable than the chronically ill or disabled, and my sense of grief was partly rooted in shame and disappointment. This bias can lead to feelings of inadequacy and failure in those of us with a wide range of visible and invisible disabilities. Ableism is cruel and absurd, as it ignores the frailty we all share. Much as we would like to pretend otherwise, we are all vulnerable to disease and disability.

For the newly disabled, acknowledging the loss of "able-bodied" status can initially feel overwhelming. Acknowledging my disability has been difficult. I have finally fully understood my complicity in unconsciously favoring the "able." Like most of us, I've been influenced by cultural and professional norms about what is expected of a contributing member of society. Though I respect those who are disabled, perhaps my view of them has been tainted by an element of pity. I now better understand the ugliness of "ableism," as none of us wants to be pitied or considered "less than." We all deserve respect as human beings simply doing the best we can.

This flare was yet another—and the most dangerous to date—reminder of the unpredictability of lupus. I had operated with an illusion of control, convincing myself that sleeping ten hours a night was enough to protect me. My worst times were when I worked excessively long hours and was sleep-deprived, so I believed avoiding this was the key to maintaining health. Despite the increased workload and other pressures, I had been getting my usual rest leading up to the flare. It was probably inadequate for my needs, though, given the situation.

We warriors know that our coworkers and employers don't understand the debilitating nature of lupus. Unfortunately, even as a physician, I found that to be true. After my major flare, one of my partners, a friend and highly knowledge-able doctor, noted that some physicians don't realize how devastating lupus can be. Another physician commented that "doctors never stop working!"—a toxic, self-destructive attitude that I no longer shared. It's important to reiterate that an ideal career for lupus patients allows flexibility, part-time options, and the opportunity for self-care.

Since lupus is an uncommon disease, not all physicians fully grasp its consequences. My rheumatologist in Cincinnati was experienced and warned me that most people with such a severe flare were never able to work again, an idea I mentally rejected. One of my other four subspecialist doctors believed I'd be able to return to work after six months, showing his lack of understanding. Even warriors in their twenties typically need at least a year to recover from such a significant flare. Another of my doctors, an older experienced, superb physician, urged me to listen to my body and rest and heal, regardless of the duration required.

It took two and a half years to recover from the flu-like feeling with this multi-organ flare, and I've never regained my baseline stamina and energy level. Even some rheumatologists, especially less experienced ones, don't fully appreciate how life-altering lupus can be. As mistaken beliefs about the disease abound, we must trust ourselves and pay attention to our bodies to protect ourselves.

We should never allow ourselves to be "gaslighted" into thinking we are lazy, unmotivated, or imagining our symptoms. Being excessively dedicated to work or fixated on finances are poor ways to maintain our health with lupus. We must be assertive in letting our doctors know how much or if we can work. Remember that none of us is indispensable in our jobs, though our egos may tell us otherwise. Only *we* must live with the consequences of downplaying or ignoring our needs.

A British survey study of over 2500 lupus patients found that only 15 percent were working full-time and 19 percent part-time.[6] Other British researchers found that the combination of the invisibility of the disease, the fluctuating condition, and the lack of understanding by employers explains why many patients are unable to work. They conclude that "more data is needed to inform workplace adjustments if individual distress and societal loss of skills are to be addressed."[7] It's heartening to see efforts underway to accommodate our variable, changing needs.

In the U.S., researchers reported that lupus is a common cause of disability, accounting for about 20 percent of all those disabled from work.[8] A Lupus Foundation of America survey reported, "55 percent of lupus patients reported a complete or partial loss of their income because they no longer are able to work full time due to complications of lupus."[9] Currently, there is increased interest in chronic debilitating illness due to long COVID, estimated to have affected at least four million Americans to date.

The Labor Department is now seeking information regarding what can be done to help keep long COVID patients in the workforce. The Assistant Secretary of Labor for Disability Employment Policy requested online dialogue from workers and employers to obtain feedback on policies to alleviate workplace challenges for this group. This effort will hopefully lead to more prospects for all of us with invisible chronic illnesses.

* * *

As my major flare was starting, Dan was in California, house hunting. His brother, who lives there, had warned him that home prices were skyrocketing and urged buying immediately, though we wouldn't be moving for more than a year. When it became apparent how ill I was, I let Dan know that I would understand if it was too much for him to cope with and if he no longer wished to marry. He was committed to me and our relationship, even when his brother-in-law previously told him of a friend who died of lupus in her forties after being abandoned by her spouse. The in-law asked Dan if he was sure he wanted to deal with my illness, and Dan had no hesitation, nor has he since.

My parents were in their eighties by then and were distraught and afraid to see me at my sickest. Four months after the onset of my severe illness, they planned to visit. Dan suggested we marry while they were in town. Maya was still resistant to accepting Dan, which would have led to a tense, unpleasant start to any marriage. Upon hearing of our wedding plans, Maya moved in with her father nearby to spend her senior year of high school. She soon reluctantly accepted it and celebrated our nuptials with us in a quiet home ceremony.

After this flare, I continued to appear ashen with very low energy, muscle and joint pain, and malaise for a few years. Friends commented that I looked as though I felt unwell. This contrasts with the often-normal appearance of lupus patients, belying the underlying symptoms. I had developed keratitis, too, a painful inflammation of the cornea in both eyes. It was severe in the right eye, leading to reactive eyelid swelling and eventual scarring of both the cornea and eyelid. So, I have a mildly chronically swollen right eyelid, concealing part of my iris, the colored part of the eye.

Additionally, I developed painless oral ulcers and a dull pressure headache and had to sit, lie down, and rest quite often. I developed a few bouts of shingles due to the immunosuppressants and started daily antivirals to prevent recurrences. As expected, given the unimaginable fatigue, mental activity was also exhausting.

Physical therapy was the first step in my recovery and made it possible for me to begin gradually walking a little. Pacing myself was more necessary than ever. For the first eighteen months, engaging in any effort for more than half an hour was brutal. My baseline conditioning was not very good, hindering my recovery. Despite the difficulties, I felt very thankful to have survived this second kidney flare with only mild loss of kidney function.

As we warriors know, lupus can be very capricious, with no obvious or consistent trigger for the day-to-day variation in symptoms. This lack of control can be maddening for us. Even as a physician, I didn't completely grasp how severely incapacitating lupus could be until my severe flare. Denial played a role, as over the years, I've had a few lupus patients who could not work. I supported their need to focus on self-care, but as humans sometimes do, I deluded myself that I would be able to work forever!

With no choice but to rest more, I also carefully began using ultraviolet light (UV) protection to help prevent lupus flares. My UV sensitivity had drastically increased along with the severity of my disease. I kept a surgical mask handy on rare occasions when I went to the grocery store, especially during flu season.

I'd been a lifelong vegetarian and became exclusively vegan after my major flare. Dan's encouragement and extensive knowledge of the plant-based diet helped me make this transition. In retirement, he became a certified instructor for the Physicians' Committee for Responsible Medicine, an international group educating the public regarding its extensive health benefits. He has presented many talks to the community on the subject. Later, I'll address more specifically the lifestyle changes I have found helpful.

The Wolf Trails
Me West

It was a relief to move to California after Maya's graduation, escaping the memories of what I'd been forced to relinquish. As Maya had always been very independent and was starting college, I knew she would be fine. I rarely went out in Cincinnati while recovering, but when at a doctor's appointment or store, I almost invariably ran into a patient asking when I was returning to work! This was very nerve-wracking and aggravated my unwarranted, unhealthy guilt about having "abandoned" my patients and partners.

In retrospect, I realize this angst did me no favors, and I strongly urge all of you to try to avoid these unhealthy reactions. Guilt has no place in coping with chronic illness, particularly lupus. Over time, I found it possible to make a life for myself even without a full-time medical practice. I slowly discovered new ways to be in the world, as a sense of purpose is necessary to maintain my zest for life. We cannot surrender who we are entirely to the burden of lupus, though there are periods when we seem to have no choice.

We moved to northern California, to a lovely, tiny town where much was accessible within five minutes of home. This was ideal as, at this point, I tended to fall asleep if I tried to drive for more than fifteen minutes, forcing me to rely on Dan for transportation for longer distances. The first thing I explored was learning Spanish online via Duolingo to be prepared to speak with Latino patients upon resuming my practice.

Though an avid reader, I often dozed off and had to lie down and rest several times a day. After about six months, I learned of a tai chi group at the local senior center, which people of any age could join. After just five to ten minutes of this gentle and simple exercise, I was short of breath and exhausted, almost fainting during an early class.

Very gradually, I increased my endurance with short walks and tai chi. Eventually, after several years, I could sometimes participate in hour-long classes on good days, sitting and taking breaks as needed. This taught me to be patient and gentle with myself to avoid discouragement. My tai chi practice was critical to my recovery and extremely healing, both mentally and physically.

Meanwhile, problems with my eyes continued. I had developed cataracts in both eyes from the prolonged high-dose steroid treatment and had lens replacement surgery. For the first time since age nine, I could discard my eyeglasses—the silver lining to this simple procedure. Despite this improvement, my severely dry eyes and keratitis (corneal inflammation) continued to worsen over time, causing frequent blurring of my vision.

Living in a small town had some advantages, as there were flexible opportunities for volunteer work that required very little time and energy. After about a year and a half, I was recruited to serve on the local community health center board. It felt wonderful to be involved with medicine again, if only peripherally. Careful balancing of my activities was required. On days I had a commitment outside the home, I was attentive to getting adequate rest. A few weekly activities gradually became possible, though I had to miss some when my health didn't permit it.

Appa passed away a year after this move. Amma began living with us for most of the year, also spending a few months with my brother and sister-in-law in Boston. Though she's fortunately healthy, the travel back and forth became too onerous, and she began living with us year-round. As we have always been close, we feel fortunate to have this time together, and Dan has welcomed Amma in his usual big-hearted way.

Due to my immunosuppression, I continued to be extremely cautious to avoid infection. During cold and flu season, I stepped up these efforts, though I still developed occasional bouts of bronchitis. Dan was sometimes irritated by my requests that he use hand sanitizer when out for a meal. As a nonmedical person, he initially interpreted it as controlling behavior but gradually understood and accepted it.

Though I'd previously worn my hair short, I let it grow to avoid possible infection at the hair salon during flu season. I no longer had any interest in coloring my hair, something I occasionally did in my late forties. For me, the potential health consequences of more chemical exposure outweigh looking younger. It felt liberating to be in casual attire all the time and forego maintaining a professional wardrobe and appearance, and I embraced it. I'd lost much of my sense of taste to chemotherapy, which improved a little with time. These losses were insignificant in the face of my survival with adequately functioning organs. I took new pride in living to sport my gray hair!

Finally, three years after the multi-organ flare, I felt well enough to attempt working a little again. Knowing I could only tolerate at most one to two hours of activity before requiring rest, I started working two hours a week. I provided internal medicine consultations for the family practice doctors at the local community health center. This was yet another advantage of being in a small town where such opportunities are available. It felt great to see patients again, but I came home very tired each time and had to lie down to rest afterward.

After about eighteen months on the two hours a week routine, I increased it to two hours twice weekly. About a month into the new schedule, I saw the ophthalmologist for increasing eye problems. Retinal swelling was detected, a new and very concerning finding. The ophthalmologist ran some tests and diagnosed me with retinal vasculitis. My vision in the affected eye was somewhat decreased and soon worsened into the range of legal blindness.

I then requested that my rheumatologist check my labs, which showed a recurrent flare of kidney disease. My immunosuppressants, gradually reduced by about half, had to be doubled again. Evidence of a flare in any organ should always lead us back to our rheumatologist to assess for other organ involvement.

My astute rheumatologist at UCSF (University of California San Francisco) informed me that other autoimmune eye diseases were often misdiagnosed as vasculitis, which requires treatment with chemotherapy. Therefore, she recommended a second opinion from an ophthalmologist at the university medical center who is highly specialized in autoimmune disease. Fortunately, he diagnosed posterior uveitis, an auto-immune inflammation of the eye's posterior chamber. It's a rare complication of lupus and does not require chemother-apy. This was one of several times in my decades with lupus that a "super-specialist" consultation has been invaluable and spared me unnecessary chemotherapy.

Concurrently, pain from the corneal inflammation wors-ened and became severe for a few months. The community cornea specialist tried many interventions to no avail, and I developed a corneal scar in the right eye. Once again, I decided to consult at UCSF, one hundred miles away. The cor-nea doctors there ordered a scleral lens for me, a specialized huge contact lens that holds a saline solution for constant irri-gation of the eyes. When I finally obtained these, I got rapid relief from the painful keratitis and partial vision correction despite the corneal scar.

The decreased vision and threat of blindness were more alarming to me than any of my previous lupus complications. I had previously cared for a patient with sarcoidosis, an auto-immune disease known to cause severe uveitis. She initially developed vision loss from uveitis in one eye and, despite the best efforts of ophthalmology, progressed to legal blindness in both. With this scary precedent, I feared the worst-case scenario—one of the pitfalls of being a patient, made worse by my experience as a physician!

As an internist, I was used to caring for individuals with organ failure. I found the prospect of kidney failure less terrifying than blindness, which would lead to a loss of independence. Loss of sight is unimaginable to those accustomed to a lifetime of vision, and I felt great anxiety. Already exhausted from over four years of worsened illness since my major flare, I was uncertain if I had the fortitude to adjust to permanent vision loss.

My family experienced this in a very visceral way, like a physical blow. Even Dan, who typically tries to hide his emotions about my setbacks, was visibly distressed. My brother and sister-in-law wept when I told them about the vision loss, my deeply caring sister-in-law exclaiming, "I hate this disease!" I did not share this setback with Maya until it was well on the way to resolution. She was in college and working part-time, and it would have been an unfair burden. My wonderful nephew and niece are busy young adults, and I also try to protect them from distressing news.

As in some other situations, people were unsure how to react to this setback and, in some cases, retreated. This was understandable, as I would have liked to flee the situation myself! Dan pointed out that as I'm a physician and tend to be stoic, some assume that I don't need emotional support. Compassion fatigue becomes a significant problem for all who care about us in dealing with chronic illness. It's a delicate balance between expressing our emotions and over-taxing people, but we patients sometimes benefit just from being heard.

The uveitis initially failed to respond to increased immunosuppressants and standard-dose intraocular or eye steroid injections. After three doses of high-dose intraocular steroid injections over eight months, it finally resolved. As topical anesthetic was used, there was little discomfort.

However, Dan was horrified during the first injection, having insisted on being there for me. The kidney flare also subsided later in the year with increased immunosuppression. This was also a tremendous relief, though it caused yet a little more decline in my kidney function.

Dan's observation:

"There is an Italian idiom 'aver fugato' which is interpreted as 'to have strength.' On this day, I really needed it. I will never forget being asked by the doctor to stand behind Niranjana to hold her head steady as she inserted what looked like a bicycle spoke into her eyeball. Yikes!

This day provides a 'sharp' reminder that managing this disease is sometimes a team effort. I wouldn't have it any other way."

After this flare resolved, I attempted to resume my little part-time work at the local community health center. The executive director had previously mentioned that the physicians found my input very helpful. She is a wonderful person with extraordinary dedication to the community, and she described lupus as "a horrible disease." Her sister-in-law, who was only forty-two, had succumbed to lupus some years ago.

As I'd been open with her about my health condition, she had shared her grave concerns about me resuming work from the start. She urged that I consider focusing on taking excellent care of myself instead of working, as she understood that lupus could be a deadly disease. I was still hopeful I could participate for at least a few hours a week since I had recovered from the uveitis and kidney flare and felt I could handle it.

Realizing I had flared while working minimal hours, she asked me to complete a form attesting to my physical capacity. I had to be capable of working eight hours a day, being on my feet for long periods, and being seated for long periods— all of which were impossible. I realized this was her way of protecting me from myself, so I gave up the idea of working for the time being.

Though disappointed, I realized my longing for work overcame my reality. The physicians asked me, if I felt up to it, to continue my monthly lectures on topics of their choice. I enjoyed this very much and was happy to oblige, health permitting.

Dealing with lupus is similar in some ways to living with a far more benign condition, such as chronic back pain. When your back is aching, you remember to do your exercises to aid recovery. In between bouts, one forgets to keep up the movements needed to keep the pain at bay.

Similarly, with lupus, I find that the somewhat better periods tempt me to stray from the strict self-care required to stave off flares. I must keep reminding myself of what's at stake. For me, this has been one of the toughest challenges of living with the disease. The human temptation to strive for the unrestricted, "normal" existence we see others enjoy is sometimes overwhelming.

Several months later, I began noticing a gradual mild increase in my chronic shortness of breath, concurrent with bad allergies. As mentioned, I have both interstitial lung disease and COPD due to lupus. I first attributed the symptoms to airway spasms, which allergies can trigger. After a few weeks, I saw a pulmonologist, and an x-ray and lung function testing revealed nothing new.

One morning soon after, the breathing difficulty became so severe that Dan took me to the emergency room. A chest x-ray was again unrevealing, but a chest CT scan showed pneumonia. Due to my immunosuppression, I had no other symptoms but a slight cough.

I was hospitalized briefly and began improving after several doses of antibiotics. We lupus patients on immunosuppressants, and our families, must remember that our medications tend to conceal or mask symptoms of infection.

So we must take even relatively mild changes in our condition seriously and be evaluated.

After completing the course of antibiotics, I began to have high fevers, up to 102, and a bronchoscopy was performed. This involves inserting a bronchoscope into the airways to sample the deep-seated microbes directly. This revealed aspergillus, a ubiquitous fungus that can cause dangerous, life-threatening infection in the immunosuppressed. The treatment for it carries significant side effects, including changes in vision and kidney function, both problem areas for me. This was another terrifying period in my illness.

Though I'd never seen a case due to its rarity, I knew aspergillosis could be rapidly fatal and difficult to treat effectively. It occurs more often in patients who have received high-dose chemotherapy, such as for bone marrow transplants. Still, one of my rheumatologists noted she had seen it in patients with my degree of immunosuppression. I was apprehensive about it, even considering going into hospice if it got severe and I was not responding to treatment.

The threat of blindness just the year prior, followed by this infection, felt unbearable. I began to feel I could no longer tolerate lupus—both complications from the disease and the treatment. I felt reasonably confident that I could survive all my prior difficulties but was uncertain this time.

Once again, my incredible loving and generous internist friend flew in from the east coast. She came to provide her moral support, be my advocate, and see the infectious disease doctor with me, as there was uncertainty about the diagnosis. I am fortunate to have a few other very dear friends who have also been tremendous sources of support over the years, one of whom encouraged me to write my story.

I took a month of medication for aspergillus, which fortunately resulted in just temporary vision changes and deterioration of kidney blood tests. Shortly after starting this medication, I required another brief hospitalization due to fainting. There was concern about the possibility of a heart rhythm disturbance which can result from the aspergillosis treatment, but it was determined to be likely due to benign medication side effects. Scans at the end of the treatment course showed the resolution of my pneumonia.

The aspergillus appeared to be a red herring and not the cause of my illness. The university infectious disease doctor very kindly provided me with a telephone second opinion consultation and was extremely helpful, as the community doctors were puzzled. The high fevers were due to lupus, though treating the dangerous possible aspergillus infection in an immunosuppressed person was wise. Although lupus can cause fevers, lupus patients, especially the immunosuppressed ones, should *always* assume fever is due to infection unless proven otherwise by our doctors.

Too much knowledge as a physician proved stressful for me once again. These days, with internet access, patients frequently search and grow either needlessly alarmed or falsely reassured about symptoms. After nearly two tough years, my will to continue to fight was diminished, something I resolved to steel myself against in the future. There's far too much to live for!

* * *

After the shock of the 2016 presidential election results, many were distraught. In our small town, a close friend started a local chapter of Indivisible, a national activist group. I promised to support her in any way possible. This was my first real foray into political work, as was the case for thousands nationwide.

This activist work mostly involved phone calls, letters, texting, and infrequent meetings. It was physically manageable and could be done on a flexible schedule. Being part of this effort increased my sense of purpose in life. We also became involved in some advocacy work for healthcare for all Californians and Medicare for all nationally.

So, my illness and disability led to a few opportunities. Another was my rediscovery of music and the violin, something I had enjoyed very much from childhood through college. During my nearly thirty years of medical school, training, and practice, I rarely played very briefly before abandoning it due to joint pain. Now, playing the violin feels incredibly healing to me, and to our amusement, one of our dogs became my biggest fan! Cosmo pranced excitedly whenever I took out the instrument and lay at my feet to listen attentively.

I was able to renew my relationship with some extended family, especially a well-loved cousin in India with whom I'd felt close since childhood. It stung to hear her say that the family in India had decided that I didn't care for them, as I didn't visit or stay in touch. An aunt, my mother's sister, asked in a wounded tone why I had never visited her since beginning my medical career. I explained that lupus and my work schedule precluded it. As they're unfamiliar with lupus, my explanation seemed to be met with some skepticism—something we patients are accustomed to! Chronic illness disrupts relationships, but opportunities to revitalize them can sometimes be seized.

Climate Refugees

"To be a human being . . . no matter in what circumstances, not to grow despondent and not to lose heart—that's what life is all about, that's its task."

– F. Dostoyevsky

Meanwhile, climate change effects were worsening in California as elsewhere, with more frequent and far more devastating wildfires. Three consecutive years of fires and resulting poor air quality in northern California caused my chronic shortness of breath to worsen, and we dejectedly decided we had to relocate. After researching and considering the options, we moved to a beautiful mid-Atlantic region with good weather and highly rated lupus and overall medical care. So, we were among the earlier climate refugees from California, and many others followed.

Necessary as the move was, it was especially tough on Dan. He reveled in California with its large contingent of tolerant and progressive people, gorgeous terrain, and ability to be outdoors all year. Though he recognized the necessity, he was more distressed than I was. He has suffered from periods of mild depression that predated our relationship. Dan had two traumatic brain injuries, one from a motorcycle crash as a young man and the second from a bicycle accident. Although head trauma can cause depression and other psychological issues, the strain of my illness has likely contributed.

Unsurprisingly, Dan's depression worsened after the move, and he blamed my health status for it in the short term. He expressed resentment towards me, though he agreed we were facing worsening air quality from the blazes. Living in that area necessitates having a "go bag" packed should one need to evacuate at a moment's notice. If it weren't for my breathing difficulties, he might have considered staying or moving to a different part of the state with a lower fire risk. Dan's sister and brother-in-law also relocated to our community six months after us, fleeing the California wildfires. This helped ease the pain of the loss of our old community, as they are loving, considerate family members, and we all care for one another.

Dan is an adventurous, active, and energetic person who bicycled thousands of miles most of his life. Much of his childhood was spent running in the woods, with many falls and broken bones along the way. He would never have pre-dicted marrying a very cautious, somewhat sheltered person. For example, in my childhood, my parents felt camping was dangerous and incomprehensible. After all, why would anyone with a perfectly good home voluntarily sleep outdoors?

Over the years, during difficult periods, I have gently told Dan that I love him very much and want him to be happy. If he believes he could have a better life without me, I am open to him changing whatever is necessary for his well-being. Like other patients, I don't want to be perceived as an unwanted obligation by my partner. Fortunately, he loves and is committed to me and has gradually begun to appreciate our beautiful new community. Due to my low energy, Dan is very kind, bearing the brunt of household duties and chores. He's also become an incredible vegan chef and loves to cook!

Shortly before the move, I discovered a telemedicine opportunity. Energy permitting, I started doing online, urgent, on-demand consults after we settled into our new home. I was delighted to find a way to continue to practice, but as it's very fatiguing, I'm careful to limit my work hours. I may be obstinate, a slow learner, or both, but I have finally accepted what I must do to survive: take breaks and rest when my mind or body requires it.

Soon after the move, I developed another bout of pneumonia. This was followed a couple of months later by a period of increased shortness of breath and a recurrent flare of kidney disease. The increased doses of immunosuppressants for the kidney flare then predisposed me to a kidney infection a couple of months later. Periods like these, with problems occurring one after another, are very exasperating and disheartening. Sometimes, I feel angry and upset that I seem unable to get a break and weary of lupus—emotions we patients can all understand. After I recognize and process my negativity, recalling all I've managed to overcome encourages me onward.

> ### Dan's comment:
>
> *"I cannot adequately convey the sense of wonder I have seeing Niranjana confront these problems. It's like fighting a wolf with a pillow. Her unbelievable strength and commitment to 'beat the beast back' is beyond enviable. Yes, I know much of the world faces endless challenges, but this is so intimate and present; her fortitude truly humbles me. The ability to face this disease every day from all directions is exhausting for all involved. That said, I can't stop 'being there' for her since her resilience strengthens my resolve to stay by her, for better or for worse."*

I suspected the fourth kidney flare probably resulted from the strain of the move and the accompanying tension at home. Fortunately, it was resolved by increasing the immunosuppressants yet again. By now, it was apparent that a recurrent organ flare eventually resulted every time the major immunosuppressant medication dose was reduced—a disappointing trend.

As with earlier moves, it took time and patience to find new doctors. I initially met a young doctor at one of the local lupus centers who was openly annoyed by my input regarding my care. I'd never experienced this, as all my previous physicians welcomed it. Other young rheumatologists have expressed that I probably know more about lupus than they do, as I've lived with it longer than some have been alive!

Returning to a different doctor at the lupus center, I found limited continuity of care. Several physicians were on staff and saw all the patients on a rotating basis, a model that wouldn't work for me, as my case is complex. Finally, I found an excellent lupus doctor on the recommendation of my highly knowledgeable nephrologist. She has had decades of experience as a professor of rheumatology and recently went into community practice. So, a university lupus specialist may not always be the best answer for our individual needs. Exploring all your local options is worthwhile.

Meanwhile, my immune system's red blood cell destruction, or hemolytic anemia, continued to be a concern. This is a rare complication of lupus, so there is limited data regarding its management. As blood markers indicated the process might be ongoing, increasing my immunosuppressants was recommended by my rheumatologist.

However, I have received differing opinions regarding this issue over the years. As my blood counts were low but stable, and the best course was unclear, I consulted out of town with a super-specialist at Johns Hopkins University Lupus Center who has dedicated her life to lupus research and treatment. She concluded that the current dose was adequate, given the stability of my anemia.

I had an annual follow-up with cardiology, as my EKG (electrocardiogram) had been abnormal for a few years. Further testing demonstrated mild heart enlargement, likely due to the high blood pressure from my chronic kidney disease. I received an alarming misdiagnosis of pulmonary hypertension based on my cardiologist's assessment of my echocardiogram (ultrasound of the heart). This is a rapidly progressive and usually fatal condition with no effective treatment. Though I grieved, I surprisingly felt I could accept and be at peace with it. As I've gone through so much, I feel prepared for the worst.

Fortunately, the official reading of the echocardiogram showed that the initial interpretation was incorrect. This reminded me that we patients should never make assumptions based on preliminary readings before final test results are available. I should have known this as a physician, but when dealing with an emotional situation, we sometimes leap to conclusions.

Like many, I am sometimes in denial and ignore problems, hoping they will resolve with more rest. On the other extreme, as I've noted, my knowledge of the worst possible outcomes and implications of specific diagnoses sometimes causes me mental anguish. Reading articles in medical journals about unfavorable statistics regarding lupus and its outcomes is discouraging, and I avoid it to some extent. Being a physician with lupus can be a razor-sharp, double-edged sword.

Overall, though, my knowledge has been far more helpful than not. For example, when meeting new physicians in California, I saw a young, inexperienced nephrologist who suggested I abruptly stop taking my high-dose immunosuppressant for the multi-organ flare. Fortunately, I knew I was nowhere near the two to three-year mark post-flare when that could be safely considered. I also realized that tapering the medication requires great caution and must occur over the course of years!

Even now, nearly ten years later, I have been unable to reduce the dose of mycophenolate without recurrent organ injury. I carefully evaluate my test results as well as the risks and benefits of treatment recommendations, which helps me avoid complications. My suggestions regarding how we patients can all be actively involved in our care will follow in the "Management" section.

Despite all these obstacles and new evidence of organ injury, I maintain my joy in life. Dan and my mother have commented over the years that they don't know how I can bear it all, as they would be inclined to give up. Relatives and friends sometimes commend me on my bravery, but as we warriors know, we can and must rise to our challenges. The ability to continue contributing to this world in some small way is gratifying. Loving relationships with family, friends, furry companions, and the violin have helped me flourish.

The Wolf and COVID-19 Collide

"We have a chance to do something extraordinary. As we head out of this pandemic we can change the world. Create a world of love. A world where we are kind to each other. A world where we are kind no matter what class, race, sexual orientation, what religion or lack of or what job we have. A world we don't judge those at the food bank because that may be us if things were just slightly different. Let love and kindness be our roadmap."

– Johnny Corn

Though epidemiologists and infectious disease doctors had warned for decades that a pandemic would occur, the life-threatening COVID-19 still took us all by surprise. It began very soon after we relocated to the mid-Atlantic. Being in a new area made it easier to isolate ourselves since we had few established connections. Along with other high-risk individuals, I thought COVID would help the average healthy person better understand the plight of the immunocompromised. We are accustomed to regularly taking precautions to avoid infection, the importance of which the rest of the world was just discovering.

It soon became apparent that the politicization of science would be disastrous. Seeing a large population segment's skepticism, denial, and rage was horrifying. After the vaccine became available, the degree of resistance and refusal was a shock. Our sometimes noxious individualism has led some to think only of themselves, with no concern for society or healthcare workers. The signs carried by some protesters in Tennessee said it all: "Sacrifice the weak—Open TN." To high-risk individuals, the cruelty of this worldview is unfathomable.

Doctors and nurses faced anger, hostility, and combativeness from patients and, at times, family members. For the first time since I was forced to quit direct patient care, I felt some relief to be practicing telehealth rather than confronting that rage. Even still, I am infrequently subjected to animosity from patients on video calls, which can be stress-inducing. Anxiety about COVID has been so great that some patients angrily demand that I prescribe antibiotics though it's inappropriate—something I refuse to do. When lupus becomes severe, we do not tolerate tension as well as when our disease is milder, and greater caution is required.

The isolation COVID-19 has imposed on many high-risk individuals makes it more challenging to maintain a sense of optimism. The pandemic deaths, effects of climate change, political instability, gun violence, wars, threats to democracy, and other daily tragedies we currently face can sometimes lead to feelings of hopelessness. Limiting news consumption may help, and even those who believe it's responsible to stay informed need occasional news breaks for our mental health. Especially during lupus flares, knowing less about the disturbing state of the world is often healthier for us patients.

One of the most challenging aspects of COVID is the added layer of difficulty it poses for my sociable, outgoing husband. Due to my immunosuppression, I had essentially no response to the vaccines. My multi-organ disease also places me at high risk, so we are still very cautious and relatively isolated to avoid infection nearly three years into the pandemic. Many healthy people with normal immunity have resumed their everyday lives despite COVID.

Our loved ones make sacrifices from love, but as we are all human, it's sometimes difficult for them. We patients certainly compromise for our family members, too, in various ways. Illness touches almost every person or their loved ones, and we must all learn to cope.

Like countless others at high risk, Dan and I often feel trapped by the situation. The pressure I have occasionally faced from him regarding his desire for us to travel together reminds me that no one, not even those closest to us, truly comprehends what it's like living with lupus. He has reluctantly accepted that I can best gauge what I can handle. I encourage Dan to do what he loves, though it is frustrating for us both that I cannot bicycle, take long hikes, or travel at will with him.

For our self-preservation, we must learn to deal with mild coercion from loved ones calmly and with clarity. Succumbing to guilt and pushing ourselves beyond safe limits can obviously make us sicker. Trying as these situations are for family, the stakes are infinitely higher for us. Even with a loving, supportive family, the journey with lupus is ours alone.

I gained a different perspective of my concerns about restricting Dan's life from a few sources, including the book *Us* by Terrence Real.[10] Real, an experienced marriage counselor, views partners as a team that should focus on what is best for *both*. Our society emphasizes personal fulfillment above all else, to the detriment of relationships. Real argues that sacrifices made for a partner offer a chance for personal growth and benefit everyone—couples, children, and society.

Our healthy friends have also found that the devastating losses from COVID have refocused their life goals. As they are mostly older and thus higher risk, they, too, have new constraints. Those of us with chronic, limiting illnesses have already learned this lesson. We are all forced to decide what we value most when options disappear. Like other high-risk individuals, we immunocompromised warriors collectively face the unpleasant reality that our lives may never return to our pre-COVID "normal."

Early this year, Amma was ill for a week, and Dan simultaneously broke his wrist in a bicycling accident. As a result, I had increased household chores and developed a three-month flare with malaise, worsened fatigue, and increased muscle and joint pain. Headaches and brain fog also developed during that period, and I was occasionally unable to think clearly, recall, or problem-solve. Fortunately, I did not develop any new organ injury with this flare. I'm careful to perform consultations only when I'm entirely lucid. Of course, we warriors must avoid tasks requiring mental clarity, including driving, when "foggy."

The latest new difficulty I'm facing is related to the poor dental health that has plagued me and others with secondary Sjogren's syndrome. As mentioned, severe dry mouth results in cavities despite excellent oral care. Dental procedures also become riskier with immunosuppression, and I've now had two episodes of bacteremia, or bacteria in the bloodstream. These resulted from dental work, despite preventive antibiotics. This is a rare complication, puzzling the experts.

I was hospitalized for the second bout. Once again, my knowledge has been both a blessing and a curse, as I'm fully aware of the potential complications resulting from bacteremia, including sepsis and organ or bone infection. I was very anxious for a couple of weeks after hospital discharge, as I realized I was at an impasse regarding future dental care.

The work required to maintain a healthy, functioning set of teeth has become potentially dangerous for me. Ignoring needed dental work can lead to more infections, too, and of course, tooth loss. My dismayed brother commented that lupus is like "whack a mole," referring to the arcade game in which a rubber mallet is used to strike moles that reappear!

As in other rare situations, I again experienced the frustration of having doctors who are dismissive or minimize patients' concerns. The infectious disease doctor at the hospital recommended that I continue with the same ineffective antibiotic prophylaxis. I was skeptical and asked several questions about this approach, which seemed illogical. I received no answers supported by science.

As mentioned, I infrequently sense being seen as an annoying patient, as my knowledge compels me to ask questions that a typical patient would not. We all have the right to feel comfortable with our treatment plan, as *we* will deal with the consequences of our healthcare decisions. Fortunately, I obtained an infectious disease consultation at another local academic center. The physician there agreed with my concerns and, after careful consideration, developed a more aggressive preventive regimen which I am hopeful will work.

Women more often experience dismissiveness, especially from male physicians, though there are terrific and empathetic doctors of both genders. Minimizing patients' problems tends to occur more frequently in complex cases when the diagnosis or treatment is not straightforward. Some doctors incorrectly assume there's no actual disease if they don't know the diagnosis. This is experienced by those with various autoimmune disorders, chronic Lyme, chronic pain syndromes, and those with long COVID. I'll discuss tips on preparing for effective office visits in the "Management" section.

During my university practice years, several older female patients, mainly minorities, complained about their treatment by a few surgical subspecialists at our institution. Their questions were ignored, and they felt disrespected. Therefore, I felt compelled to speak to the head of the department involved, who wanted to be informed of any problems. He was very concerned and immediately rectified the situation.

We doctors sometimes use hurtful speech. A lack of empathy can be painful and anxiety-provoking for us patients, leaving us feeling alone in coping with our condition. In her eloquent memoir about her experience with chronic illness, Meghan O'Rourke notes that a physician she saw told her she'd rather have cancer than chronic illness.[11] The reasoning was that you either recover or die with cancer, implying the physician would rather die than live with chronic disease. There was likely no malice behind the statement, just a lack of consideration.

This exemplifies the inadequate training in communication and sensitivity we physicians may receive. Temperamentally, we humans also have differing capacities for compassion. I observed that residents and medical students have vastly disparate bedside manners. For some, the skill comes more naturally than others, and not every trainee seemed to appreciate its importance. Physicians who habitually use upsetting language may be best avoided.

Currently, I am still more fatigued and symptomatic with lupus than I was ten years ago, before my major flare. I have gained some strength over the past two years by utilizing most of my daily energy "allotment" on walking and a little yoga or tai chi. Work and other activities are secondary, as improving my fitness and health are essential to give me the needed reserve to cope with recurrent flares. I hope to remain independent rather than require nursing home care in the future. I give thanks each day for what I'm able to do and continue to nurture my passion for life!

Healthcare Inequities and Lupus

"The top 1 percent have the best houses, the best educations, the best doctors, and the best lifestyles, but there is one thing that money doesn't seem to have bought: an understanding that their fate is bound up with how the other 99 percent live."

– Joseph E. Stiglitz, The Price of Inequality: How Today's Divided Society Endangers Our Future

". . . the true measure of any society can be found in how it treats its most vulnerable members."

– Mahatma Gandhi

Healthcare and societal inequities disproportionately impact lupus patients, other chronically ill, the indigent, and the elderly. Unequal access to care adversely affects us all, as tax-payers pay emergency care costs for the uninsured. Healthcare costs are a leading cause of bankruptcy in our country, even for the insured. Our highly flawed healthcare system is why we are ranked the lowest among wealthy nations in health outcomes, despite spending far more money per capita. Life expectancy in the U.S. ranks below more than sixty other countries, according to the World Bank.[12]

A recent survey of eleven wealthy countries again placed us last in healthcare outcomes.[13] We ranked lowest in access to care, life expectancy, and maternal and infant mortality. Those who cannot afford regular office visits wait until they are critically ill and go to the emergency room, so we also have the highest preventable death rate due to a lack of timely care delivery. COVID-19 made inequality in care even more apparent, as Blacks and Latinos were hospitalized and died at significantly higher rates than White Americans. Only recently has this trend reversed with more deaths in White Americans, believed to result from lack of vaccination. Additionally, in 2021, more than half of Americans have postponed or foregone medical services for financial reasons.[14]

Even pre-COVID, there have always been significant disparities based on race and ethnicity. Minorities, the poor, and rural Americans utilize healthcare less than other groups due to its availability and expense. Thus, they have the poorest outcomes in rates of illness and death. According to the Centers for Disease Control, "Across the country, racial and ethnic minority populations experience higher rates of poor health and disease in a range of health conditions . . ." Black Americans' life expectancy is four years less than that of white Americans. Lack of care access may partly explain why minorities suffer from more severe lupus.

The U.S. is the only wealthy, industrialized country that does not provide healthcare for all. Twelve percent of adults in the U.S. are uninsured, and another 21 percent are underinsured. Furthermore, many of us believe that exorbitant costs in our for-profit system are grossly unjust in our prosperous nation. According to the Bureau of Labor and Statistics, in the past twenty years, individuals' out-of-pocket healthcare expenses have more than doubled, while median income has only risen about 55 percent.

Physicians for a National Health Plan is among multiple groups that have advocated for universal healthcare since the 1980s. More than 20,000 physician members, like me, support coverage for all. Many of my patients, including the insured, struggle to buy their medications, as the pharmaceutical industry charges far more for the same drugs here than in other countries.

Maintaining employment can be very difficult for lupus patients, so the model of employer-provided health insurance is especially problematic. Loss of insurance and medication access is a genuine risk for those with lupus, as for other chronically ill and disabled patients. For example, an older, legally blind woman with a kind and radiant spirit shared her increased troubles in the wintertime. She was forced to choose between buying her medications and heating her home. She loved to dance and joked that it helped her stay warm despite the cold.

Like other caregivers, I was able to call the power company. If a patient's condition meets the company's definition of "medical necessity," gas and electricity are supplied for a month. Many older people on a fixed income share her difficulties. With climate change causing more extreme weather, conditions are becoming more hazardous for the elderly and chronically ill.

Clearly, calling the power company is only a temporary fix, and the bills eventually come due. Like healthcare, heat is a necessity for everyone living in cold climates, not a privilege only the well-to-do should have. Some cities like Baltimore are piloting projects in cooperation with local medical centers to house the homeless, recognizing that deprivation has a devastating effect on health.

For example, one winter month on hospital ward duty, I saw a diabetic patient repeatedly intentionally overdose on his diabetes pills. He wanted to be hospitalized to come in from the cold—a risky ploy that fortunately did not kill him. Social services placed him in a homeless shelter each time, but he felt unsafe there, sadly preferring the noisy hospital.

Ideally, as in other wealthy countries, our U.S. healthcare system should provide this basic need we all share. However, increasingly and unjustly, it functions as a for-profit business. This trend started in the 1970s and 1980s and has spiraled out of control, especially with the consolidation of hospitals leading to monopolies.

Private, religiously affiliated, and even some "public" hospitals frequently focus on profits over patients. Those working in public hospitals occasionally receive indigent patients transferred from private emergency rooms. They are told that "you'll get better care there" after performing the so-called "wallet biopsy." However, federal funding is provided to *all* hospitals to care for the needy.

Lobbying Congress by lucrative specialists' groups has kept reimbursements very high, and there's no billing standardization. Even some specialists have been critical of their fellow providers for excessive use of procedures. They point out that primary care doctors (including internal medicine, family medicine, pediatrics, and obstetrics/gynecology) provide far more cost-effective care. The Affordable Care Act has provided a partial solution, though twelve states have currently refused to expand Medicaid, the federal health insurance plan for low-income individuals.

Furthermore, many private practice offices do not accept Medicaid, so access to care is even more limited. My husband was shocked to learn this and called many private doctor's offices in Cincinnati to investigate. None of the many he contacted accepted Medicaid. If you are on Medicaid, look for care at a local academic or university medical center, if available. Many medical school faculty accept Medicaid, as my group did at the university. If the faculty don't accept it, locate the hospital fellows' clinic, where doctors who are training in rheumatology often see patients with the supervision and consultation of faculty physicians.

If you cannot access good lupus care from a rheumatologist where you live, seriously consider relocating, though the pain and fatigue of lupus complicate this. If you are uninsured and in a state that did not expand Medicaid eligibility, moving to a state with better Medicaid access can improve your overall health. In the U.S., "grandfathered" health insurance plans still exist, which can refuse coverage based on pre-existing conditions or exceeding lifetime benefits. However, marketplace plans can no longer do so, thanks to the Affordable Care Act.[15]

If there are medications that are recommended and financially out of your reach, call the drug manufacturer. Pharmaceutical companies will occasionally provide free medication for the needy. The Lupus Foundation of America is a fantastic nonprofit organization that recently posted a list of financial assistance resources, found at https://www. lupus.org/resources/financial-assistance. This site provides resources for assistance with medication, medical and dental care, mental health care, housing, and much more. If you're not yet on their mailing list, sign up, as they provide a wealth of information. For struggling, low-income patients with lupus and other chronic illnesses, researching possible pro bono financial counseling sources is also worthwhile.[16]

Even with optimal self-care, lupus flares can still occur. Those more fortunate can take the necessary steps to stay healthy, such as cutting back or quitting working when needed to rest and recuperate. Unhappily, these options are unavailable to many. In this regard, a lovely lupus patient comes to mind, who developed blood clots in her legs that posed a risk of gangrene.

Fortunately, she did well, and amputation was not necessary. She was in her thirties and recovered after a few years from that flare and began working for one of the largest low-cost national retailers. In those days, they enforced mandatory overtime, which exhausted her, threatening her health.

I wrote her employer a note stating that she must be exempted from forced overtime due to her medical condition. They ignored my recommendation, causing her more joint pain, fatigue, and worsening of her condition. In their new employee orientation, the employers demonstrated the process of applying for Medicaid, as they relied on part-time employees to avoid paying for health insurance. Unfortunately, many businesses use this strategy.

An additional problem is that worsening and unjust income inequality makes it impossible for many to save enough to alter work schedules to attend to their own or a family member's health. It is distressing and infuriating to see patients grapple with physically demanding minimum wage jobs such as maintenance who are too ill to work but unable to obtain disability. Often, applying multiple times and obtaining the assistance of a disability lawyer can be effective. So, if you cannot work due to your chronic illness and are denied, try again. Hopefully, we will someday live in a more just society that values and cares for all of us.

PART TWO

Keeping the Wolf at Bay: Management Guide

"In the middle of this road, we call our life
I found myself in a dark wood
With no clear path through"

– Dante Alighieri

So, you've been diagnosed with lupus and are wondering what to do now. These practical considerations are instrumental in helping those living with lupus. I will delve into what I've found useful and what's recommended.

Preventive measures may help you achieve remission and stave off organ-injuring flares. Best of all, the side effects of prevention are all beneficial, as they are health-enhancing! Once lupus becomes severe, as I'm experiencing, the chances of remission diminish tremendously. A crucial point worth repeating, we warriors must *constantly* prioritize what is health-promoting!

Rest, Rest, Rest!

We Americans are a sleep-deprived society, and according to the CDC, "Insufficient sleep is a public health epidemic." Sleep deprivation affects learning, memory, attention, mood, etc., even in the healthy. Rest is critical for lupus warriors; we typically need far more than healthy people.

With lupus, sleep deprivation is potentially dangerous! Carefully listen to your body, and rest when fatigued. Ten hours or more of sleep a night is typical for lupus patients, and most of us also require a nap to avoid exhaustion. Daytime naps should be limited to one hour, if possible. Staying awake after 3:00 p.m. each day helps to prevent insomnia. Adequate rest reduces symptoms of fatigue, muscle, and joint pain.

Maintaining and adhering to a rest schedule while adjusting for daily fluctuations is essential. For example, having to awaken even thirty minutes earlier than usual or a disrupted afternoon rest can cause increased symptoms. Your need for rest can change over time, depending on disease activity, so you must always remain keen observers of your state of health.

Inadequate rest, as well as overactivity, can aggravate systemic inflammation and increase autoimmune activity. Stress hormones, including cortisol and epinephrine, are activated, increasing inflammation and disease activity. These hormones also injure heart health, causing increased blood pressure, heart rate, and blood sugar.

Immobilization during periods of extra rest requirements increases one's risk for potentially fatal blood clots, so keep your legs moving frequently. As some of us with lupus have antibodies predisposing us to thrombosis (clots), this movement is even more essential. Flexing and extending the ankles, like stepping on and off a gas pedal, helps prevent clots. When traveling for long periods, use this technique as well. Incidentally, be very cautious when driving since fatigue makes us more prone to falling asleep behind the wheel.

Though we require rest, we warriors of all ages sometimes struggle to sleep. Some note insomnia is more problematic during flares. Pain, depression, anxiety, and higher-dose steroid treatment can be factors, and a vicious cycle can develop. Poor sleep, pain, and fatigue make it difficult to function the next day. The resultant inactivity can aggravate muscular pain, as worsening muscle weakness makes us more prone to strain and spasms.

Staying in bed or being inactive during the day further compromises sleep, as getting at least some exercise is essential to good quality rest. Guard against excessive bedrest and remaining bed-bound even during flares. In addition to weakness, immobilization predisposes you to obesity, diabetes, cardiovascular disease, worsening osteoporosis, and more, so some activity is necessary.

Good sleep hygiene can significantly improve sleep quality. These measures include avoiding caffeinated products such as coffee, tea, sodas, energy drinks, and chocolate (especially dark) after noontime. Some individuals are excessively caffeine sensitive and must eliminate it entirely to sleep well. Avoid light-emitting devices like phones or computers for at least one hour before bedtime, as they trick your brain into thinking it's daytime. Your body then fails to produce natural melatonin, which causes drowsiness. It's also best to keep bedroom clocks turned away and avoid checking the time overnight, as the resulting anxiety can worsen insomnia.

Vigorous exercise should be avoided for a couple of hours before sleep, as it's stimulating. A soothing, regular bedtime routine such as reading, quiet reflection, or a warm bath or shower improves sleep. Relaxation techniques, including progressive muscle relaxation, can be helpful and are available on YouTube. Specific coping strategies will be addressed later, which further promote quality sleep.

A cool temperature and complete darkness in the bedroom are helpful. Some find white noise useful, especially in noisier urban environments. The bedroom should be reserved for sleep or intimacy only, as engaging in other activities creates an association with mental stimulation.

Maintaining a regular sleep schedule is best, though the variability of your symptoms can interfere. For those having sleep issues despite these lifestyle measures, consider a cognitive behavioral therapy program specializing in chronic insomnia. The Society of Behavioral Sleep Medicine offers a list of practitioners to help you locate providers in your area.

Remember that self-medicating is problematic. Alcohol is a poor choice as a sleep aid, producing poor-quality, frequently disrupted sleep. Sleeping medications can cause side effects, including dependency, drowsiness, and injuries, and are best avoided.

Sleep deprivation from nocturnal hot flashes can be an additional problem for post-menopausal women with lupus. I spent decades hearing my older women patients complain of having to fling off and put on their bedsheets at night, and then later experienced it myself! For some unlucky women, hot flashes continue for many years. After age fifty, your circadian rhythms are altered and your sleep patterns change for the worse. It becomes harder to get into the deeper REM (rapid eye movement) sleep stages, so awakening occurs more often than in the young.

Simple lifestyle measures reduce hot flashes, including lowering room temperature and using fans. Wearing layers of clothing and light layers of bedding that can be shed helps. Avoid triggers such as stress and spicy foods. Lupus warriors are generally not good candidates for estrogen hormone replacement therapy, as estrogen can trigger lupus flares. Soy in the diet, certain antidepressants, and other medications can relieve hot flashes, so speak with your doctor about these safer alternatives.

Exercise

Regular exercise is essential to dealing with lupus. It's worth reemphasizing that we must resist the temptation to lie in bed all day when exhausted and in pain! Exercise is proven to help combat lupus fatigue. Though some lupus doctors suggest increasing doses or adding new immunosuppressants to treat fatigue, this approach may be riskier.

Exercise has added benefits of increasing fitness, reducing stress, improving mood, and helping one maintain independence. As physical therapists observe, "Motion is lotion," increasing strength, mobility, and reducing pain. A recent medical journal review confirmed the safety and benefits of exercise for lupus patients, including improved quality of life and reduced risk for heart disease.[17]

We warriors must attain the highest fitness level possible. Take advantage of better periods to do so, to build some reserve for more difficult times. After a flare, especially a major one, we are often weakened and deconditioned, and poor fitness impairs recovery. Remember that in most circumstances, it's possible gradually to regain strength with physical therapy, patience, and perseverance.

Walking is an excellent pursuit if you've been inactive. Start gradually and aim for at least thirty minutes daily. The day-to-day variation in exercise tolerance is a problematic, tricky aspect of life with lupus. It's like walking on a moving tightrope, but your ability to assess appropriate activity levels improves somewhat with experience. Remember, too, that moving as much as possible throughout the day has been proven beneficial in several studies, lowering body fat, blood sugar, and cholesterol. This frequent movement should occur along with the daily minimum half-hour exercise.

The best exercise is one you will do consistently and won't be too hard on your joints. Running is usually not a good choice, as it can trigger joint pain and swelling. My favorite is walking, and I also try to incorporate some gentle yoga and tai chi daily. The meditative aspects of both these exercises is very therapeutic; both are profoundly relaxing and gratifying.

In tai chi, one must practice mindfulness and be in the present moment to focus one's attention on the next pose. As my insightful tai chi teacher and friend notes, this helps us tap into our "natural state of contentment." Many studies show the health benefits of tai chi for numerous ailments, ranging from arthritis, chronic pain, depression, to heart and lung disease.[18]

Qi gong, the tai chi warm-up exercises, are soothing range of motion movements that maintain flexibility. These are available on the internet if attending a class is not possible. Yoga also has health benefits, with studies suggesting improvements in hypertension, chronic pain, certain auto-immune diseases, depression, anxiety, and more.[19]

The balance work in tai chi and yoga is crucial for those with osteoporosis induced by steroids, often used in lupus treatment. Hip fracture confers a high risk of long-term disability and is a leading cause of nursing home placement in older adults. Loren Fishman, M.D., of Columbia University, has developed a "yoga for osteoporosis" video available online, which was found to be effective in increasing bone density.[20] Three different levels of difficulty of the poses are provided so that anyone can find the right fit. Working with a yoga teacher can help prevent injuries and is a good idea for beginners.

Remember that weight-bearing exercise is best for osteoporosis. Simply put, it is exercise that requires you to be on your feet, supporting the weight of your body. Therefore, swimming and biking have less effect than other choices. Movement may sometimes cause acute (i.e., new onset) inflammation of joints, for which rest, ice, and elevation are helpful and may avert the need for more medications. When pain or swelling prohibits weight-bearing exercise, other options like bicycling can maintain muscle strength. Those with osteoporosis may consider using an exercise bike rather than bicycling outdoors, as falls and fractures can be averted.

Pain Management

Pain is universal in lupus patients but variable in severity. Joints, muscles, and connective tissues are the primary sites affected, and headaches are also common. Some of us may develop bone pain due to osteoporotic fractures or avascular necrosis of the hip. The latter condition is the death of bone tissue and can occur in those who have received high-dose steroids. If the pain is severe, it is treated by hip joint replacement surgery.

We lupus patients tend to assume all our pain is from our disease. However, there can be other underlying conditions. Your doctor can best make this determination. Osteoarthritis may contribute to joint pain in older lupus patients and can be alleviated by physical therapy. Vitamin D deficiency and hypothyroidism can also cause musculoskeletal pain, and both are easily assessed by blood testing.

If you suffer from whole-body pain, talk with your doctor about fibromyalgia, to which we patients are more prone. Fibromyalgia is a non-inflammatory chronic pain syndrome involving primarily muscles and connective tissues, with associated sleep disturbance and fatigue. Medications such as statins used to treat high cholesterol can also cause muscle pain that occurs symmetrically, i.e., involving the same areas on both sides of the body.

Remember that although lupus can cause headaches, a multitude of conditions of the eyes, ears, sinuses, teeth, blood vessels, etc., can also do so. A thorough examination and evaluation are needed. Tension headaches are more common due to the stress of lupus, and those with a family history of migraine headaches or cluster headaches may suffer with these. Targeted treatment for your specific condition is important, so do not assume lupus is the culprit.

If other factors have been excluded and your pain is due to lupus, speak with your doctor about the best management approach. *Avoid self-medicating!* Some over-the-counter medications may be unsafe for you or may interact with your prescriptions. For example, if you are on steroids, taking over-the-counter ibuprofen or similar medications raises the risk of gastrointestinal bleeding significantly.

Achieving a good balance between proper rest and exercise along with Plaquenil is adequate for many patients. Ice for acute (recent onset) musculoskeletal pain, heat for more chronic (longstanding) pain, and massage can be helpful modalities to improve your pain control. Some may find acupuncture helpful. For those with severe refractory or uncontrolled pain, a multi-disciplinary clinic specializing in pain management may be beneficial. Later, coping emotionally with chronic disease will be discussed, as sound psychological health tends to alleviate pain.

UV Protection

Our understanding of the role of UV protection in lupus management has evolved over the decades, as simply wearing a hat was previously recommended. Now, we know that regular clothing affords only a very low level of UV protection. UVA and UVB lights, present in sunlight and tanning beds, activate the immune system in lupus, and many of us notice that we feel worse after UV exposure.

Some of us also develop rashes, or photosensitivity, from sun exposure. Even if you haven't developed rashes or other symptoms, avoiding UV light (including halogen and fluorescent lighting) is still important in staying healthy with lupus. Remember that even when it is cloudy, there is UV light present. Unless it is dark outside, protection is needed year-round.

The current recommendation for lupus is to use sunscreen with an SPF of at least fifty-five. Remember that you need a thick, visible coating with "physical" sunscreens for effectiveness. These contain zinc oxide or titanium dioxide and have the advantage of not being absorbed into the bloodstream. The protection can be patchy, however, as the barrier minerals may be unevenly distributed in the product.

The chemical blockers, which don't contain zinc or titanium, are more effective and can be rubbed into the skin. However, they can be absorbed into the bloodstream, and some of these may increase the risk of non-skin cancers. Studies show chemical sunscreens reduce the risk of melanoma, the most dangerous skin cancer, so dermatologists continue to recommend them. All sunscreens require periodic reapplication if you remain outdoors for more extended periods, so the directions must be carefully followed.

Consumer Reports tests various sunscreen options so that you can rely on their findings, as the FDA does not study or regulate these products.[21] Other protective options include UV barrier clothing, hats, and umbrellas. Limiting time outdoors between 10:00 a.m. and 4:00 p.m. and staying in shaded areas also reduce your exposure.

I find the UV umbrella plus SPF clothing simpler to use than sunscreen, and these newer options are now more widely available. Adding a UV protectant film to car windows reduces the symptoms we may experience after being in the car. Wearing sunscreen or SPF clothing and a hat in the car adds extra protection—especially worthwhile for longer journeys. Some find their UV sensitivity increases along with disease severity, but prevention is worthwhile for all lupus warriors.

Diet

Healthy eating is essential for lupus patients and avoiding processed (packaged) and fast foods is vital. The excessive salt, sugar, and fat usually found in these foods are undesirable for anyone, but even more detrimental for us. In addition, processed foods often contain ingredients that could be lupus triggers. A good rule of thumb is to put the package back on the shelf if you don't recognize all the labeled components. Much is unknown about the vast array of chemicals we are bombarded with, and whole foods are our safest choice. Selecting organic foods is best for the same reason, as pesticides may trigger immune activity.

Casein, a protein found in dairy products, has been identified as inflammatory, and some experts consider a plant-based diet to be the least problematic. The China Study, by Cornell's Dr. Colin Campbell, is worth reading for those who would be open to considering this diet. Appendix one provides a list of selected resources for more information on the whole food plant-based (WFPBD) diet. Physicians nationwide are increasingly recommending the vegan (WFPBD) diet for the health benefits across the board.

The plant-based diet is associated with reductions in diabetes, heart disease, and cancer. After age fifty, cardiovascular disease is a leading cause of death in lupus patients. Three decades ago, cardiologist Dean Ornish, M.D., demonstrated the reversal of coronary artery disease with a plant-based diet.[22] It's taken a long time to gain traction, as our eating habits are deeply ingrained. Many physicians are reluctant to change their own. The WFPBD is nutritionally richer than a standard American diet (ironically known as SAD!), though a vitamin B 12 supplement is essential.

Researching the vegan diet carefully to obtain all the needed nutrients and consulting your physician are important. Daily consumption of leafy greens and legumes, such as soy, black beans, garbanzo beans, or lentils is advisable. For those who develop gas from beans, soaking them overnight and discarding the water is one effective method of reducing the gas-forming sugars. Our bodies adapt to bean consumption and the problem subsides naturally over time.

If going plant-based seems impossible to you and your family, simply incorporating more vegetables, fruits, and legumes (beans and lentils) into your diet and reducing your intake of animal products is helpful. Even eliminating dairy can reduce symptoms. Anecdotally, one of my lupus doctors recommended eating more kale to me, as he's seen several patients feel better while consuming it daily. It packs a tremendous nutritional punch and has anti-inflammatory and antioxidant effects. Eating a colorful and varied array of vegetables and fruits ensures better nutrition.

There is growing interest in our microbiome, or the multitude of bacteria in our gastrointestinal tract, referred to as our intestinal flora. Plant foods improve the composition of the flora and promote "good" microbes. In contrast, processed foods and artificial ingredients are harmful and can adversely affect the immune system, increasing the risk of chronic diseases.[23] Fermented foods such as yogurt (non-dairy and dairy), kimchi, kefir, tempeh, and kombucha tea help propagate plentiful "good" bacteria in our intestines, reducing inflammation.

Some researchers suggest aiming for at least thirty plant foods daily, which is more achievable than it sounds. Spices and herbs are an excellent way to increase your daily intake, for example, by adding small amounts of cinnamon, cardamom, and cloves to your morning oatmeal. Light (steeped briefly to reduce caffeine content) green or white tea with ginger has anti-inflammatory and antioxidant effects, reducing cardiovascular and cancer risks. Incorporating various ethnic foods into our diets adds many spices and is delicious!

A recent British online survey was conducted of lupus patients placed on a more plant-based diet with increased vegetables and decreased sugar, processed foods, and dairy. The researchers found that 80 percent of these patients reported feeling significantly better with this simple change.[24] They experienced fewer constitutional symptoms like fatigue, pain, and improved mood. Reducing dairy had the most significant effect.

An additional advantage to a plant-based diet is avoiding antibiotics overused in the meat industry. According to the FDA, at least 70 percent of antibiotics used in the U.S. are for meat production. These can potentially lead to more resistant or difficult-to-treat infections, to which immunosuppressed warriors are more prone. The situation is becoming increasingly dangerous as bacteria are "outsmarting" our available antibiotic options. Chicken and meat intake are associated with highly resistant bacterial infections in humans, for example.[25,26]

Avoid garlic and especially alfalfa sprouts, as these activate the immune system.[27] Anecdotally, some find that nightshade vegetables like potato, eggplant, and tomato may worsen symptoms, so you may want to experiment with eliminating these. In the past, nutrition textbooks warned that psoralen-containing foods including parsley and parsnips can be photosensitizing, but there is no evidence to support this. Be alert for any foods which you notice trigger your symptoms.

Omega-3 fatty acids may be helpful and are found in walnuts, flaxseed, chia seeds, and fish oil. Note that flaxseed should be ground for optimal absorption and can be sprinkled on cereal, salads, yoghurt, etc.

There's no hard evidence that turmeric is effective, but some lupus patients report feeling better using it. Its efficacy is tremendously boosted by combining it with black pepper, which is contained in some supplements. Talk to your doctor first before trying turmeric, as it may increase bleeding risk when taken in combination with medications having a blood thinning effect, such as aspirin. There are also recent rare reports of turmeric-induced liver failure.

During a flare, weight loss tends to occur, and caloric intake should be increased. Obtaining nutrients through a well-balanced diet is far better than taking supplements, as you get fiber and more nutritional value overall. If you're concerned that you're not eating well, adding a multivitamin may help.

To promote bone health, adequate calcium intake is essential. It's best to get calcium through your diet, and Appendix two provides a list of common food sources. Calcium tablets can be constipating and cause kidney stones. These supplements can also deposit in arteries, predisposing to atherosclerosis, with coronary artery disease possibly resulting.

Talk with your doctor about how much calcium you require, as it varies by age and the condition of your bones. If you cannot get enough throughout the day, take a supplement with eight ounces of water to flush it through the kidneys to make up the difference. Your doctor can tell you whether calcium carbonate or citrate is best for you based on your health status and medications.

Vitamin D is also traditionally considered essential for bone health, and those deficient may suffer from musculoskeletal pain. Lupus experts believe adequate vitamin D levels may protect patients against autoimmune disease activity;[28] therefore, blood levels over 40-50 ng/mL are suggested by many rheumatologists. We warriors must monitor our levels and take vitamin D3 supplements as recommended by our doctors. A recent New England Journal of Medicine study raised doubt about the effectiveness of vitamin D in preventing fractures in healthy adults,[29] which does not apply to lupus patients. Osteoporosis experts continue to recommend vitamin D3.

If you have kidney disease, talk with your nephrologist about any dietary restrictions needed. With hypertension secondary to kidney disease, salt restriction is required. A low salt diet is generally advisable in lupus patients, as the steroids we may require cause salt retention, elevating blood pressure and cardiac risk. Avoid taking *any* over-the-counter medication without your nephrologist's approval. Pain medications like ibuprofen and naproxen are especially injurious to the kidneys, raise blood pressure, and must be avoided by everyone with even mild kidney disease.

With advanced kidney disease, potassium intake must be restricted as the kidneys don't appropriately excrete it. High levels can lead to heart rhythm disturbances which can be life-threatening. Salt substitutes should be avoided, as they usually contain potassium. The same is true of magnesium-containing products, so be cautious with supplements or seemingly innocuous medications such as milk of magnesia. Protein intake may also need to be adjusted, as a high intake can aggravate severe kidney failure. Some nephrologists recommend limiting protein even with less severe kidney disease, which is still controversial, so speak with your nephrologist.

Substance Use: Tobacco, Alcohol, and Cannabis

We will now turn to the need to guard against falling into substance use or abuse to deal with stress. Some of us with addictive personalities and a family history of alcoholism are more prone to this. It can stealthily overtake anyone, so be on the alert. There are excellent reasons for lupus patients to avoid these habits beyond the serious health problems they can cause.

Tobacco

Smoking in lupus patients increases autoimmune activity, leading to poorer health outcomes. Recent evidence shows an increased incidence of lupus developing in smokers, and tobacco decreases the effectiveness of Plaquenil, an essential cornerstone of lupus therapy.[30] Also, smoking is one of the significant risk factors for cardiovascular disease. Both chronic inflammation in lupus and steroids used in treatment tend to clog arteries.

Furthermore, lung disease can result from smoking, aggravating injury we may already have from our disease. Immunocompromise and smoking make us more prone to lung infections and scarring. These are just a few of the many adverse effects of tobacco, including multiple cancers. It's well known that lung cancer is associated with smoking. Fewer are aware that many other cancers, including those of the head, neck, esophagus, pancreas, kidney, and bladder, are linked to smoking.

Lupus is associated with an increased risk of lung cancer, even in nonsmokers.[31] If you require a C.T. scan of the chest, ask your doctor whether a low radiation dose scan rather than a standard scan might be appropriate to reduce your exposure. Lupus warriors must quit smoking!

Alcohol

In general, alcohol can be toxic to many organs, including the liver, heart, pancreas, brain, and peripheral nervous system. As lupus can damage your organs, why add a potentially harmful substance? Alcohol raises the risk for a multitude of cancers, including those of the head, neck, esophagus, and liver. As lupus patients tend to have impaired immunity and the need for immunosuppressants can further predispose us to cancer, drinking compounds the hazards.

In addition, alcohol can cause gastritis (stomach inflammation) and gastrointestinal bleeding. Certain medications we may require, including steroids, can also increase the likelihood of these complications. Adding alcohol to many medicines is risky business.

You have probably heard that red wine protects against heart disease. Reservatrol, the protective substance, is also found in red grapes and grape juice. These are far safer ways to enhance your heart health. That said, a rare glass of wine or champagne on a special occasion should not be harmful to those who are not in recovery from alcoholism.

Cannabis (Marijuana)

Now that cannabis use is widespread and legal in most U.S. states, it's worth mentioning. Risks may include heart and lung problems, psychosis, and suicide. It causes impaired attention and concentration and, in some cases, causes motor vehicle accidents. The cognitive problems lupus patients sometimes experience are aggravated by cannabis. Lung cancer risk may increase with its use. As we lupus warriors already face many health challenges, we are wise to steer clear of it.

Medical Care

Remember, lupus is very unpredictable, and it's important to keep all your appointments. The capricious and erratic wolf can creep up on us! Typically, you should see your rheumatologist at least every three months. However, for those with milder lupus and no organ problems, every six months may be adequate if recommended by your doctor.

It's so important I'll repeat the critical point that you must remain vigilant, watch for changes, and be seen if exhaustion, new, unusual, or flare symptoms occur. Also, monitor yourself for decreased appetite or unintended weight loss of more than a few pounds. Always err on the side of caution and be evaluated if in doubt. Remember, too, that the diminished mental clarity that may accompany flares can make it difficult for you to assess the situation. Your family should be made aware of this potential and be alert for changes you might have overlooked when it comes to getting needed medical attention.

We doctors are human, and things can rarely be missed, so monitoring your test results is helpful. Be proactive in your care and request and review your lab results. Ask about any abnormalities, especially in your urine studies, which should be regularly checked. Blood in the urine should generally not be attributed to menstruation in women and requires follow-up. Over the decades, I have rarely been the only one to notice a new kidney flare based on my urine results.

Keep a file of your medical records, focusing on test results. All radiologic imaging reports and biopsy results are essential. Antibody test results verifying your diagnosis and routine lab results can help your physicians, especially if your various subspecialists don't share a medical record system. Changing doctors when needed is easier with this information in hand.

Although individualized to each patient, a urinalysis and urine protein/creatinine study should generally be done every three months, per rheumatologists. Kidney function, liver function, complete blood counts, and C3 and C4 are typically monitored. The latter two are indicators of autoimmune activity, and when they are lower than expected may indicate an impending organ flare.

Be aware that even with normal inflammatory markers (ESR and CRP), we may feel poorly, though it would be unusual to develop significant organ injury. Many rheumatologists do not monitor these due to the lack of correlation with the disease activity. Lupus does not follow the textbooks, and each case is different! I had very high inflammatory markers for the first twenty-eight years of my condition but relatively mild symptoms for much of that time. Since my severe flare ten years ago, I have had periods of feeling poorly despite normal ESR and CRP levels.

Remember that lupus is an enigma even to rheumatologists, as there is minimal data on treating uncommon complications. There can be disagreements about the best approach, even with common ones like kidney disease. Consulting super-specialists who focus on lupus treatment and research, usually found at university medical centers, can sometimes be helpful for diagnostic or treatment dilemmas.

Ideally, seek a doctor who is experienced, knowledgeable about lupus, listens well, and responds to your concerns. Evaluating potential doctors' credentials, years of experience, and online reviews are helpful. If you know others who see a doctor, learning about their experience is valuable. Compassionate care is desirable, but knowledge is most important. Be sure your doctor is accessible to you when you're ill and urgently need help. You need a doctor who is your advocate and supports your need for medical leave, if necessary.

Some techniques to help with doctor's visits include having a list of your medications, symptoms, concerns, and questions in order to avoid forgetting. Taking deep breaths before an appointment can be helpful if you are anxious. Accompaniment by a friend or family member may provide moral support. Tenacity about having your needs addressed before leaving the office is helpful.

Also, see an internal medicine physician (internist) at least yearly. There are qualified family doctors; however, they receive far less training in adult medicine, as they also practice pediatrics and obstetrics/gynecology. Since lupus patients are often medically complex, an internist may be a better choice.

Maintaining routine preventive care, including cancer screening, is essential and should be regularly reviewed. Subspecialists are knowledgeable in their field, but your primary care doctor specializes in prevention, monitoring, and coordinating your overall care. Studies show that chronically ill patients often miss recommended preventive care appointments because we are so busy with specialist visits—a pitfall to avoid.

Medications

Compliance with medications is critical for all lupus patients. The half-life of some drugs (which predicts how long therapeutic levels remain in your body) is relatively short, so missing doses can reduce effectiveness. Experts agree that Plaquenil should generally be taken by all lupus patients who tolerate it, which is rarely a problem. It is proven to reduce symptoms of fatigue, malaise, pain, and rashes. There is evidence that it may prevent flares, thrombotic (clotting) problems, and reduce organ damage. Plaquenil enables the reduction of steroid doses, and a few researchers have suggested that it may increase life expectancy.[32]

Plaquenil suppresses disease activity, though you won't feel any noticeable effect when taking it. I've had lupus patients who stop it because they don't experience the burst of energy they do with steroids. Once they understand the importance and take it as prescribed, patients invariably feel better. If the dosing is appropriate for your body weight, it's extremely rare to have any retinal (eye) issues, and current testing detects changes early enough to prevent permanent damage. The current recommended dose is a maximum of 5 mg of plaquenil for each kilogram (2.2 pounds) of a patient's bodyweight. A yearly exam with an ophthalmologist is critical to screen for problems.

Prednisone and other steroids, in general, should be used as sparingly as possible, as the side effects are serious. They include suppression of immunity, atherosclerosis (predisposing to heart attacks and strokes), hypertension, diabetes, weak muscles, osteoporosis, cataracts, glaucoma, and more. High doses are infrequently necessary for prolonged periods during a severe flare, but rheumatologists are aggressive about tapering them off when safely possible. *Do not self-medicate!* I have seen patients who take steroids on their own when feeling poorly, a dangerous practice.

Do not reduce steroid doses on your own, either, as adrenal hormone fluctuations can occur, causing weakness, fainting, and other symptoms. Selected patients require a low dose chronically, and you should talk to your doctor about your case. If once-daily dosing is recommended for you, it's best to take it around 8 a.m. with breakfast to simulate your body's production of cortisol, your natural corticosteroid. Other immunosuppressants are often used to reduce steroid doses in those with difficulty tapering off them. We all know that steroids in higher doses increase the appetite, add unwanted weight, and produce sugar cravings. Increased blood sugar and diabetes mellitus can then result.

Knowing whether the dose of steroids you require suppresses your immune system and makes you more prone to infections is helpful. Very low doses do not affect immunity significantly but can help constitutional symptoms like fatigue and pain. Keep track of dose changes; you must take extra precautions against infection on higher doses. If you require emergency care, be sure the treating doctors are aware if you are currently on steroids or if you have taken them in the past year, as this information enables them to guard against potentially dangerous adrenal hormonal fluctuations.

When there is organ injury, more potent immunosuppressants are typically required to decrease your immune system's attack on the body, and chemotherapy may be necessary for certain severe complications. Many lupus experts believe that only organ involvement can justify immunosuppressant drug use. They believe the risk of infection, cancer, and other side effects of the various drugs may outweigh the benefits of using them for non-life-threatening symptoms. Recall that adding more immunosuppressant medication as well as increasing doses raises the risk of side effects but is sometimes necessary to preserve the function of vital organs.

Ask your doctor about the risks and benefits of proposed new medications and whether current research supports adding them. It is crucial to avoid delays in treatment with active, ongoing organ damage. A second opinion is reasonable to consider if in doubt about the need for immunosuppresant drugs, increasing doses, or adding new drugs. Remember, too, that these medications must generally be continued for at least a few years after any organ damage has stabilized.

Also, as a general rule, it may be wise to avoid medications that have been out for less than three to four years unless there is no good alternative. In the first few years after a drug is released, unanticipated and sometimes serious adverse effects may be seen.

Be aware of drug-induced lupus, typically a milder form of the disease that can occur due to the development of autoantibodies on certain medications. It may be seen after months or even years on medication and resolves within a few months of discontinuing the offending drug. Procainamide, hydralazine, and minocycline are among the most common causes, though several other drugs have been implicated. Check with your doctor about whether any of your medications might be responsible for or contributing to your symptoms.

Certain drugs and supplements can cause lupus flares, including sulfa drugs such as Bactrim,[33] often used to treat urinary infections. The immune system stimulant echinacea can cause flares and must be avoided, and some experts believe melatonin may also be problematic. You may want to keep this list handy as many doctors may be unfamiliar with these potential hazards. Remind your doctors to help you avoid medications that may cause photosensitivity (increased sensitivity to sunlight), potentially worsening the disease activity.

Keep a list of medications and doses in your purse or wallet, with generic and brand names. Keep this updated, including any supplements, and be sure your partner or family knows where it is in case of emergencies. Be informed about the purpose of each of your medications and review them on your visits. Using a pill organizer helps prevent forgotten doses, which can occur as we often take drugs more than once daily. If traveling, be sure to have an extra supply of medication in case of unanticipated delays in returning home.

Avoid looking for "miracle" cures or drugs being peddled on the internet, as well as charlatans who claim they have all the answers. Unless they have randomized, controlled, double-blinded trials with data to back up their claims, conventional medicine is the safest route to good lupus care. Alternative treatments may have dangerous side effects or interact with prescription medications in unpredictable ways.

Secondary Sjogren's Syndrome

Some with lupus also have secondary Sjogren's. As noted, this primarily causes autoimmune destruction of the lacrimal or tear glands and the salivary glands, causing dry eyes and mouth. Primary Sjogren's occurs without another associated autoimmune disease and can cause symptoms including fatigue, rashes, joint pain, and swelling. It can also lead to kidney and lung disease.

Dry Eyes

Dry eyes can feel gritty, painful, and cause the sensation that something is in the eye. With untreated or severe eye inflammation, corneal abrasions, ulcers, and vision loss can result. I'll review treatment options, having dealt with this for decades and found that ophthalmologists are not always familiar with them. A simple test called a Schirmer's test by an ophthalmologist can determine the severity of your condition.

The first step with milder dry eyes is artificial tears. If you need lubrication more than a few times a day, the preservative-free tears must be used, as the preservative in the bottled tears can cause redness and irritation. There is a wide variety of preservative-free tears, and newer versions also contain an oily flaxseed component to better simulate tears. It takes some experimentation to determine which type works best for you. Lubricant ointment applied inside the lower eyelids at bedtime can be beneficial, particularly if you have discomfort or pain on awakening.

Your general ophthalmologist will often perform punctal occlusion, blocking the ducts that drain the tears you produce to keep them around longer. Topical drop formulations of immunosuppressants may be helpful, though some people find them very irritating to the eyes and ineffective. Prescription hydroxypropyl cellulose ophthalmic inserts (Lacriserts), which provide relief for up to a full day, can be highly effective and reduce the need for artificial tears. Twice daily, warm compresses to the eyelids with moist or dry heat for ten minutes per application are also recommended for dry eyes. If you have moderate to severe dry eyes and inadequate symptom relief with your regimen, consider seeing an ophthalmologist specializing in the cornea.

Serum tears are sometimes used for more severe dry eyes; some find this soothing. Your blood is drawn, and the serum is extracted and used to lubricate your eyes. You may need steroid eye drops if you develop keratitis or corneal inflammation due to dry eyes. It's essential to keep up with regular ophthalmologist monitoring when using steroid drops, as they predispose to cataracts and glaucoma. In more severe cases, scleral lenses, oversized contact lenses that hold saline and require a unique insertion technique, provide significant relief.

Occlusive eyeglasses and sunglasses block air exposure and prevent drying, and they are beneficial outdoors. If you suffer from allergies, these can also alleviate the resulting eye irritation. Avoiding wind or direct fan exposure is helpful. Be aware that the eyes can become more inflamed with lupus flares, and keep up with lubrication, even when feeling poorly. See your ophthalmologist for eye pain, vision changes of any kind, and annual Plaquenil evaluation.

Dry Mouth

Saliva provides an essential buffer to acid, so dry mouth leads to cavities, even with excellent care. Some medications we may take can aggravate dry mouth. Ask for your dentist's and hygienist's recommendations on an aggressive preventive regimen and toothpaste to reduce your risk of cavities, and follow it. Soft bristle brushes and very light pressure on the teeth are recommended to prevent damage. If your dentist recommends brushing after meals and your schedule makes it impossible, at least rinse your mouth thoroughly with water.

Use caution with toothpaste, as most now have whiteners that are abrasive to teeth. Find out if you're a good candidate for prescription fluoride toothpaste. Discuss water flosser use in addition to regular flossing with your dentist, especially if you have gum disease. Ask if you may benefit from a night-guard, which is helpful for bruxism (grinding) and generally maintaining gum, tooth, and jaw health.

Avoiding sweets, including fruit juices, is imperative for those with dry mouths. Fresh fruit is nutritious and accept-able for our teeth, but the concentrated sugar in beverages is harmful. Sticky foods, including dried fruit, can also be prob-lematic. Carbonated drinks are acidic, destroying enamel and causing caries. Even carbonated water is mildly acidic and best avoided. Some dentists recommend drinking water in one sitting instead of sipping, as water washes out what little saliva we produce, and it takes about twenty minutes to regenerate. Snacking has the same effect, and dentists recommend against it.

Xylitol is a plant-derived sugar alcohol, and a high xylitol content chewing gum recently recommended for me by my dentist. It's been shown to reduce cavities in high-risk indi-viduals.[34] Sugar-free xylitol gum and candies, especially sour ones, tend to stimulate the secretion of saliva. This is worth considering with your dentist's guidance if you're having recurrent problems with your teeth.

If you are taking certain osteoporosis medications or they have been recommended, it's helpful first to ensure your dental health is good. See your dentist before starting these medications to have any needed work performed. Rare but serious adverse effects are more likely with extractions or other procedures when taking these medications. An association has been reported between osteoporosis and molar tooth loss,[35] yet another reason for aggressive preventive care and seeing a dentist every six months.

Maintaining good dental health is even more critical because we may require immunosuppressants, which raise the risk of dental procedures. Research and find a dentist you can trust who will work with you on prevention rather than procedure driven. If dental care is too expensive for you, investigate your local community centers' dental services. Be aware that some private dentists will also offer free or discounted care, so ask your local providers. Local dental schools are another potential source of affordable care.

As my dentist noted, you'll get five different opinions if you see five dentists! Ask for a second opinion if many procedures are being recommended. Obtain specifics including the risks and benefits, and consider doing your own research. If you are immunosuppressed, talk with your doctor and dentist about whether you should consider prophylactic antibiotics for dental procedures. The immunosuppressed warrior should also speak with their doctor and dentist about prophylaxis if they have foreign bodies, such as artificial joints that could become infected. Anecdotally, I'm aware of patients who have developed such infections.

Longstanding dry mouth can lead to loss of taste and tongue and mouth burning. Increased sensitivity to acidic foods, spicy foods, and mint products, including mint toothpaste, can develop as a result. There are specific kinds of toothpaste (such as Sensodyne) and fluoride rinses (such as Closys) designed for those with sensitive mouths. When we're feeling poorly and struggling to keep up with all the demands of our lives, it can be daunting to invest the extra care required due to dry mouth. It's well worth it in the long run, however.

Prevention of Heart Disease

It's increasingly recognized that the inflammation accompanying certain autoimmune diseases is a significant risk factor for cardiovascular disease. Vascular disease encompasses coronary artery disease leading to heart attacks, cerebrovascular disease leading to strokes, and peripheral vascular disease leading to poor limb circulation. Compared to age-matched controls, adult lupus patients of all ages have a far higher rate of heart attacks, a leading cause of death in lupus warriors. Therefore, you must be particularly aggressive in managing your risk factors for heart disease.

The other main risk factors for cardiovascular disease include hyperlipidemia (high cholesterol), hypertension (high blood pressure), diabetes mellitus, and smoking. If you are a male over forty-five or a female who is over fifty-five or post-menopausal, your risk is also higher. Early heart disease in one's family, defined as having a first-degree male relative with cardiovascular disease at age fifty-five or younger or a female relative at age sixty-five or younger, increases one's risk. Obesity, inactivity, and a diet lacking vegetables and fruits all predispose to atherosclerosis, the narrowing of arteries leading to heart attacks and strokes. Regular monitoring of cholesterol profiles and blood sugar is essential, following the recommendations of your internist.

Many of us have high blood pressure due to kidney disease or medications, and it must be well-controlled. A home digital blood pressure monitor like the Omron should be used at least monthly for home monitoring. It should be checked and recorded for your doctor more often during periods when the pressure is running higher than desirable. The typical goal is less than 130/80, but some experts recommend that lupus patients' blood pressure goal should be less than 120/80 given our elevated cardiac risk. Speak with your physician about your personal target.

Raynaud's Phenomenon

Many of us experience Raynaud's, an uncomfortable or painful sensation in the fingers usually triggered by cold exposure. There may be associated color changes, with a classic tricolor response of white to blue to red fingertips. This is due to intermittent constriction or narrowing of the arteries in our fingers. Wearing multiple layers in cold weather and covering as much of the body surface as possible, including gloves and a hat, help prevent it. Two layers of gloves and socks are helpful in colder climates.

Emotional stress can also trigger Raynaud's, and avoiding smoking is critical to prevent it from worsening. Severe cases can rarely lead to gangrene and loss of fingers. If you have Raynaud's, it's helpful to verify with your doctor that none of your medications could aggravate the problem by constricting your arteries and reducing blood flow. Raynaud's is not believed to correlate with lupus flares, though some of us warriors notice it happens more when we're flaring. Medications that dilate the arteries are available to treat it if lifestyle measures alone don't work.

Family Planning

Decisions regarding reproductive healthcare are more complicated for female lupus warriors. There are several layers of complexity, as birth control pills (hormonal contraception) with estrogen can aggravate lupus depending on the disease's activity. Hence, you should discuss this with your rheumatologist. Consider other nonhormonal options, such as an intrauterine device or IUD, with the help of your gynecologist.

In addition, some of us have antibodies predisposing us to blood clots, making certain types of birth control even riskier, as they, too, increase clot risk. Your rheumatologist routinely screens for these antibodies, and you should understand your results, as they can also raise the risk of miscarriage. Neonatal congenital heart problems can rarely result from specific autoantibodies produced by some with lupus. If you have a history of blood clots, be aware that estrogen should not be used, as it drastically increases the recurrence rate.

We should consider pregnancy only after our disease has been very quiescent or relatively inactive for at least six months, as lupus flares can result from pregnancy. If you have organ damage such as kidney involvement, the risk increases, and consultation with a high-risk obstetrician is essential. Planning is critical, especially in this era of severe restrictions on women's reproductive rights. As there's a genetic link, our children may develop lupus or rheumatoid arthritis, and clusters of the two diseases are sometimes seen in families.

Having children is a highly personal decision, but it's essential to consider your disease, overall life situation, and whether you can safely manage one or more children without undue risk to your health and survival. These general considerations apply to warriors of all genders. Whether we will and must continue working is a factor, as this alone can consume all our energy. Maternal sleep deprivation is a given during early childhood and is more problematic for lupus patients. A highly supportive partner and family members can be health-preserving. Also, ensuring affordable childcare access and sound support systems are even more important than for the healthy parent, as we may need more assistance.

Immunosuppression

We immunosuppressed (immunocompromised) lupus warriors face unique challenges in addition to what's been mentioned. Plaquenil is an immunomodulator and does *not* increase the risk of infection as other lupus medications do. Monitor yourself for symptoms of infection, including respiratory symptoms, urinary, gastrointestinal, and skin.

A body temperature of 101.5 or greater has a higher likelihood of resulting from a bacterial rather than viral infection and requires immediate attention. To reiterate this critical point, remember that immunosuppressants tend to mask signs of infection, and we may not run a fever as a healthy person does. Those over sixty-five also have more subtle symptoms when infected due to an age-related decline in immunity. If bedridden, take several deep breaths periodically to keep the alveoli or tiny air sacs in the lungs expanded. The collapse of the alveoli predisposes one to pneumonia.

If you are started on immunosuppressants by your doctor, it is often for a major organ flare. Learn the recommended duration of treatment, when it may be safe to begin tapering or gradually reducing the dosage, and the typical time course for the taper. This way, if you move or see another physician who is less familiar with lupus, you can avert a recurrent flare. Be aware, too, that more frequent lab monitoring may be recommended when immunosuppressants are reduced, and follow through meticulously.

We must take all recommended vaccines and remember that "live" vaccines containing living microbes are unsafe while taking immunosuppressant medications. The Centers for Disease Control website provides up-to-date information on current immunization guidelines. As many of us have an inadequate response to COVID vaccines, talk with your doctor about whether there is any effective preventive antibody treatment available. EVUSHELD, previously used in the immunocompromised, is believed to be ineffective against newer variants.

Also, speak with your doctor about whether you should discontinue your immunosuppressant drugs for one week after the COVID vaccine to enable your immune system to mount a response. *Never stop your medications on your own!* Remember, N-95 and KN-95 masks are the most effective against COVID-19, and we should use them if possible when there's the potential for exposure. As some fraudulent mask manufacturers exist, look for "NIOSH," indicating government certification of efficacy.

Travel is difficult for lupus warriors, as it's arduous even for the healthy. The schedule disruption, adjusting to possible time zone changes, and the temptation to overdo it can lead to exhaustion. The immunosuppressed must remember the additional risks of infection, especially when traveling to developing countries where food and water may be contaminated with a higher frequency than in the U.S. Talk with your doctor about whether preventive antibiotics or vaccines are needed if leaving the country. Check the Centers for Disease Control website on the food and water precautions required for any overseas destination.

We also need to be aware of food recalls in the U.S., as bacterial contamination of food rarely occurs here, too. Raw produce, especially greens such as spinach and romaine, as well as raspberries, are a few that have had problems. As cooking spinach enhances nutrient absorption, this is preferable and safer. Raw, unpasteurized dairy products and even *pasteurized* soft cheeses can cause listeriosis, a dangerous infection in the immunocompromised, pregnant, and elderly.

Listeria is less commonly found in other foods, including raw fish and raw sprouts. Cooking thoroughly or avoiding these is safest. Heating foods until steaming or the internal temperature is at least 165 degrees Fahrenheit kills listeria. Packaged foods like peanut butter, deli meats, and even produce rarely carry listeria, so it's helpful to stay abreast of the news. Everyone should practice careful kitchen hygiene. Non-vegetarians must be especially fastidious in sanitizing their kitchens thoroughly, as animal products more often harbor bacteria.

If you are immunosuppressed and hospitalized with an infection, remember to ask the doctors at the hospital to consult with an infectious disease specialist, as rare conditions can occur. Infectious disease physician input can at times be helpful even if you're treated as an outpatient. Consultation with a rheumatologist about your immunosuppressant medications is also essential if hospitalized. In some situations, the most potent immunosuppressant(s) may need to be temporarily discontinued to allow your immune system to fight the infection. Your doctors will weigh the risks and benefits and make this decision.

Coping

Everything can be taken from a man but one thing: the last of the human freedoms—to choose one's attitude in any given set of circumstances, to choose one's way."

— V. Frankl

Losses in lupus and other chronic illnesses are multifold. We contend with physical limitations with repercussions in every aspect of our lives. Our ability to function as family members and in other relationships is affected. Work capacity can be affected, creating financial pressures, and interfering with our identity and purpose. We mourn these losses while wrestling with our physical challenges.

Addressing chronic illness with calmness and clarity is necessary for our mental well-being. Given the mind-body connection, a positive outlook dramatically enhances physical health and very likely our chance of survival. We've all observed that during periods of stress or excessive fatigue, even the healthy are more prone to medical problems, ranging from minor viral infections to heart attacks. Advances in neuroimmunology have demonstrated the damaging effects of stress on the immune system. These include impaired resistance to infection or cancer, and possible activation of autoimmune illness.[36]

How do we cope with lupus? Living with a chronic illness, especially one as uncertain as lupus, causes emotional turmoil and is always humbling. Especially during significant flares or new organ problems, one tends to experience a wide spectrum of feelings, including denial, shock, sorrow, anxiety, frustration, discouragement, anger, fear, confusion, despair, and finally, acceptance. The stages and emotions experienced are similar to Elizabeth Kubler-Ross' description of confronting death, as a blow to our health brings our mortality to the forefront. Along with love, joy, beauty, and wonder, it all makes up the messy, rich, complex patchwork of our lives.

Complicating matters, depression and anxiety can accompany chronic lupus and flares of the disease. Addressing and treating these is integral to optimizing physical health. Counseling can be invaluable! Sparing our family and friends from the brunt of our emotions is better for all of us, and an objective listener can provide insights or resources we may have overlooked. Therapists sometimes use a helpful analogy. When we have a rock in our shoe, we immediately remove it, and we do the same with unpleasant feelings. Naming and identifying our emotions diminish their impact, but many of us are not taught this skill in childhood and must practice it consciously.

Unjust as it is, mental health services are inaccessible for many. If you have a place of worship with psychological support sources, don't hesitate to call on them. Lupus support groups can be invaluable, as we can relate to and provide comfort to one another. Consult with your physician about antidepressant medication, which can be helpful if other options fail.

We warriors have all witnessed the toll lupus takes on our family members. It increases demands upon them and imposes restrictions. Like us, they are frightened by the uncertainty and would like to ignore or avoid it, wishing it weren't so. It's difficult for our family to know how to best support us, as our symptoms vary daily and sometimes even hour to hour. They experience chronic tension due to the unpredictability of our situation. My healthy eighty-seven-year-old mother often fears losing me—a hard loss for any parent, though I'm over sixty years old! Counseling and support groups can benefit those living with us.

Here's Dan's viewpoint:

"So, how do I handle this brutal disease daily? Firstly, with gratitude that I can be here for her. I know the challenges

won't ever be easy, but my love for this woman is boundless. Secondly, recognizing that, even for a very capable, experienced physician, there will be surprises, and some alacrity is needed. Thirdly, I remind myself that this situation could be far, far worse, and we are fortunate to be in a place where we can usually manage the disruptions this beast lays out for us. Finally, though I know that resentment for lupus interfering with MY needs can rear its ugly head occasionally, I remind myself to look inward and strive to be the best person I can be for this lovely fellow traveler."

As I've alluded to, my insight into the resilience of the human spirit gained from work has convinced me that we warriors can handle living with lupus. The grace and dignity of a young mother comforting her beautiful toddler daughter afflicted with fatal inoperable brain cancer, glioblastoma multiforme, is an unforgettable image from my medical school days. Children's unquestioning acceptance of what life brings is an inspiration for adults. I witnessed joy and laughter in children with leukemia, some of whom would not survive their illnesses.

A few of my patients suffered from rare, unremitting, and extremely painful neurologic disorders, and their courage was astounding. I saw several young people die of lupus, AIDS, and other diseases in the eighties and early nineties before more treatment options became available. These experiences reinforce the fragility of health and life and remind us to cherish each day Fortunately, untimely deaths occur less often with our expanded medication arsenal.

Discarding beliefs about what we "should" be doing is critical for our peace of mind. Though it's painful, all of us with lupus and similarly debilitating chronic illness must learn to let go of what is no longer realistic. It can be a lengthy process to achieve this acceptance and contentment despite our limitations. We must focus on and celebrate what we *can* do while maintaining the best possible health. Adapting to the need for career changes or modifications can be difficult or even heartbreaking.

The grief of losing a valued career is never gone, like losing a loved one. Nearly ten years after giving up my academic practice and teaching, its intensity still surprises me when it unexpectedly strikes. I cried when asked if I missed my academic career during a recent doctor's appointment. Though survival must now be my primary goal, the pain of loss doesn't disappear.

Please don't lose hope, though, as we can truly reinvent ourselves in this age of frequent job changes and opting out of the workplace. Being forced to go part-time or to a less stressful or physically demanding job is best viewed as an opening to explore other interests and allow time essential for self-care. Approaching necessary changes positively has served me very well, and will hopefully work for you.

There is an element of entitlement in our difficulty accepting diseases and other distressing situations in our lives. Living comfortably in the affluent western world and witnessing very little poverty spoils many of us. We expect our path to be perfectly smooth. Buddha observed nearly 3000 years ago that life entails suffering for everyone—even the healthy.

I'm still honing my ability to cope and simply sharing some options and what helps me. When I've congratulated myself on my ability to handle whatever lupus throws at me, a new wrinkle appears—a new or recurrent organ injury or a potentially dangerous infection—and it's clear it was a mirage. Anxiety surges until the new challenge or loss can be processed. Coming to terms with our mortality is daunting, as the primitive brain's survival instinct rages into high gear. Acknowledging death as a natural part of life requires wisdom that eases all our journeys.

Some Coping Strategies

These are some stress-reduction techniques that we can utilize without formal counseling. What we choose to focus on develops neural pathways, causing these thoughts to become recurrent. It's beneficial to remind ourselves that our anxiety and thoughts are *not* reality and redirect ourselves to positive self-messaging. Chronic illness makes it easy to fall prey to ruminating on worries and imagining the worst. Obsessing about the past and harboring anxieties about the future also rob us of our tranquility. We can actively choose to avoid this trap of the "monkey mind," which constantly scampers around.

Being present with mindfulness practice reminds us that this is the only moment we can be sure of, given the tenuous nature of life. We can learn to observe our thoughts, recognize their passing nature, and discover our peaceful, calm core by focusing on our breath. Mindfulness can improve our capacity to deal with negative emotions. It raises our confidence to handle whatever life presents with equanimity, or calmness and composure.

Reducing stress this way is excellent preventive medicine. Some are intimidated by meditation practices, concerned that they're not doing it right, or incapable of sitting still. It is well worth exploring, and several free phone apps, including Headspace and Insight Timer, can get you started, walking you through the process.

The origins of mindfulness meditation lie in Buddhism and Hinduism, though it's not a religious practice per se. Due to the health benefits, it's now utilized by many top U.S. medical centers. Psychologist Jon Kabat-Zinn, Ph.D., pioneered a stress reduction clinic at the University of Massachusetts Medical Center in the 1970s. He used meditation and yoga to help patients with illness, pain, and stress.

More than 25,000 have completed Kabat-Zinn's eight-week program with success, reporting significant reductions in their symptoms at the conclusion. Participants also noted improvement in their stress tolerance.[37] The University of Massachusetts offers weekly online sessions in these relaxation techniques. Kabat-Zinn's book "Wherever you go, there you are" is a lovely and insightful introduction to his methods and mindfulness practice.

Practicing compassion towards ourselves can be very salutary and reduce our stress levels. Most of us are compassionate towards family members and friends but very self-critical. Self-soothing involves actively sending ourselves encouragement and comfort. Nurturing ourselves helps us achieve acceptance and forgiveness for our often-diminished physical capacities. Placing one's hand on the heart is suggested by Zen Buddhist teacher Thich Nhat Hanh to boost the effectiveness of this practice. Hanh recommends smiling first thing in the morning, which studies confirm improves our mood.

A regular gratitude practice is essential for me and is proven to increase happiness and contentment. This can be written or more informal. For example, when starting and ending each day, I find it *transformative* to ponder all the reasons to give thanks. My personal list is headed by life itself and the ability to breathe and see—basics that my disease has threatened. It continues to include my organ function, the love of family and friends, and more. This practice can also focus on a few events each day for which we are thankful.

Gratitude must extend to our ailing bodies, too. We who are chronically ill and those with chronic pain syndromes may perceive our bodies as betraying us. This can lead to counterproductive hostility and anger toward our bodies. This stress can aggravate the disease or painful condition, and redirection to healing thoughts is beneficial and relaxing. Appreciation aimed at the body and sending curative thoughts to our cells, tissues, organs, and organ systems can deepen our thankfulness and reduce harmful tension. Adding positive affirmations and visualizing ourselves as healthy, strong, and healed may also prove helpful.

Other health and happiness-promoting habits include connecting with others, as increasing evidence demonstrates. Those with strong social connections live happier, healthier, and even longer lives! Lupus makes maintaining ties more challenging due to unpredictability and low energy. We should avoid allowing fatigue to cause withdrawal from loved ones.

Support from family and friends is essential, and extended family and friend support lightens the burden on household members. Those friends who are worth keeping will understand and accommodate our needs, something I've found repeatedly in my life. The old cliché "a friend in need is a friend indeed" holds true; some will be with us for the long haul.

Our loved ones should realize that we patients benefit greatly from relationships that are *mutually* supportive. Family and friends are at times fearful of burdening us as we already have problems. However, we genuinely appreciate those who respect us by sharing their own lives and issues, allowing us the chance to care for them, too. Like everyone, we want to contribute, rather than merely being objects of pity. Refusing to wallow in our own troubles uplifts and empowers us.

Coping is further enhanced by spirituality. Researchers at the Mayo Clinic concluded, "Most studies have shown that religious involvement and spirituality are associated with better health outcomes, including greater longevity, coping skills, and health-related quality of life (even during terminal illness) and less anxiety, depression, and suicide. Several studies have shown that addressing the patient's spiritual needs may enhance recovery from illness."[38] Part of the equation here is likely fostering connection, as religious people are more likely to be immersed in a faith community.

Spirituality, in general, is beneficial to those with chronic illnesses. Different individuals have their concepts of the term; for some, it may be religion and God-focused. For others, it may refer to a sense of unity and connection with others and the universe. The common element seems to be a deeply meaningful inner experience that touches the core of one's being. Prayer is calming and relaxing; many without formal religious affiliation turn to it for comfort.

For some, spirituality may involve mindfulness practice/ meditation, as some participants in mindfulness programs report it was the most spiritual experience of their lives. Others view their work as a deeply meaningful or spiritual calling. This is often the case for those who work in social justice movements, activism, politics, teaching, healthcare, music, the arts, or whatever their passion may be. A variety of experiences enabling one to pursue meaning and personal growth can profoundly enrich us.

Furthermore, pets are a great emotional comfort, and at least some studies have shown human benefits, including lowering blood pressure, heart rate, and stress hormone levels. Dog ownership and the walking it fosters benefit our mental and physical health. Animals' pure joy in little pleasures is uplifting, and they constantly remind us that to love and be loved is an essential element in life.

Additionally, spending time outdoors daily for as little as ten to twenty minutes is reported to have emotional and health benefits. Any natural setting will do, and for decades, the Japanese have recognized its value and encouraged "forest bathing" (Shinrin-Yoku) or simply being in a natural environment. Absorbing your senses fully in the moment by seeing, smelling, and hearing your surroundings augments the value. Walking in my neighborhood with my dog is one of my greatest, simple pleasures. Small delights are treasured more when facing physical limitations.

Energy permitting, we should make time each day to do what we love. For those of us who value mental pursuits over physical activities, travel, or adventure, our bodily constraints are easier to accept. I encourage lupus warriors forced to give up their favorite sports or other strenuous activities to seek new sources of satisfaction and fulfillment.

Openness to exploring new ways of life and novel activities is critical. Artistic or creative work can replenish, so let's experiment with the unfamiliar. My retired brother-in-law, an accountant and avid surfer, for example, discovered a love of quilting and needlepoint, much to the family's surprise. His beautiful works of art now adorn all our homes.

Research demonstrates that we can all cultivate the capacity for optimism and happiness. Nobel prize-winning writer Rabindranath Tagore observed a century ago that "everything that belongs to us comes to us if we create the capacity to receive it." The longest-running study of happiness is the Harvard Study of Adult Development. Looking at over 700 people for decades, they found that letting go of past failures and paying attention to and doing what makes you happy is effective. They also confirmed that staying connected to family and friends and developing a sense of purpose is integral to happiness or contentment.[39]

A British Medical Journal study showed the benefits of volunteering in bringing purpose and increasing our happiness.[40] The time and exertion involved may be impractical for us warriors, but even small random acts of kindness add to our sense of well-being. Studies repeatedly show that people grow happier as they age, reflecting partly a *choice* to make the fewer remaining years as positive as possible. Maybe we learn not to worry about minor issues from a lifetime of experience.

Our culture encourages the fallacy that wealth and status are necessary for happiness, but studies show that people in all socioeconomic groups report being happy. Rejecting the societal drive towards constant entertainment, stimulation, and frenetic activity is health-promoting for those with lupus. We can all cultivate a sense of contentment, regardless of our limitations or material possessions. Laurie Santos, Ph.D., of Yale University, offers a rave-reviewed free online course on Coursera entitled "The Science of Well Being" with techniques to increase our happiness.[41]

Life with lupus and other chronic illnesses can entail grueling challenges, but we can grow in response. Some psychologists have observed that the happiest people are often those who have overcome suffering to find meaning in their lives. In *Man's Search for Meaning*, Holocaust survivor and psychiatrist Viktor Frankl described his joy in the beauty of nature when imprisoned, affirming life despite the hardships of the concentration camp. Frankl noted that the Nazis took every possible freedom from their captives. However, the prisoners maintained the liberty to control their attitudes and responses to their circumstances. Some individuals rose above adversity to help others in any way possible, actually finding significance and purpose in a horrific situation.

Despite the abundance of advice about finding happiness, it remains a personal effort. Psychologists have pointed out that some may find that the various strategies make us feel worse if they fail to help us, as we are all different.[42] As I've found with my writing, journaling your experiences may be therapeutic. Ultimately, each of us must summon our ability to cope with and accept life with lupus—work no one else can do for us. Losing the will to live impacts our survival, and we must guard against this.

I have fought and clawed my way out of the hopelessness sometimes induced by life with lupus, as we patients all struggle to do. Each new challenge we face reinforces and builds our strength and wisdom to carry on. We are adaptable and must embrace our lives and change what's necessary to heal and thrive. Including joy and laughter each day, if possible, balances the heavy weight of illness. In this one precious life of ours, may each of us find some measure of inner peace.

Connect with Niranjana:

website: http://lupusinthejawsofthewolf.com
email: LupusWolfJaws@gmail.com

Appendix 1: Selected General Resources

Note: This is not a comprehensive list, and additional resources can be found via the internet. Please note that contact information for these entities may not be current and must be verified.

Patient Advocacy Groups

American Association of Kidney Patients

https://aakp.org/

American Autoimmune Related Diseases Association

https://autoimmune.org/

American Kidney Fund

https://www.kidneyfund.org/

Arthritis Australia

https://arthritisaustralia.com.au/types-of-arthritis/lupus-systemic-lupus-erythematosus/

Arthritis Foundation

https://www.arthritis.org/

Arthritis New Zealand

https://www.arthritis.org.nz/

Looms for Lupus

https://looms4lupus.org/

Lupus and Allied Diseases Association, Inc. (LADA)

https://www.ladainc.org/

Lupus Canada

https://www.lupuscanada.org/

Lupus Europe

https://www.lupus-europe.org/

Lupus Foundation of America, Inc.

https://www.lupus.org/about-us/contact-us

Lupus U.K.

https://www.lupusuk.org.uk/

National Kidney Foundation

https://www.kidney.org/

National Osteoporosis Foundation

https://www.bonehealthandosteoporosis.org/contact-us/

Sjögren's Foundation

https://www.sjogrens.org/

Professional Organizations

American Academy of Dermatology

https://www.aad.org/

American College of Rheumatology

https://www.rheumatology.org/

U.S. Government Resources

Centers for Disease Control and Prevention

https://www.cdc.gov/cdc-info/index.html

CDC Chronic Kidney Disease Initiative

https://www.cdc.gov/kidneydisease/index.html

Department of Health and Human Services Online Resources

https://health.gov/myhealthfinder

National Institute of Arthritis and Musculoskeletal and Skin Diseases

https://www.niams.nih.gov/

National Institute of Diabetes and Digestive and Kidney Diseases

https://www.niddk.nih.gov/

National Institutes of Health

https://www.nih.gov/

Social Security Administration

https://www.ssa.gov/agency/contact/

Lupus Support Groups

Inspire: Lupus Connect Support Group

https://www.inspire.com/groups/lupusconnect/

Kaleidoscope Fighting Lupus

https://kaleidoscopefightinglupus.org/

Lupus Research Alliance

https://www.lupusresearch.org/

Lupus Warriors

https://www.facebook.com/lupuswarrior

My Lupus Team

https://www.mylupusteam.com/

Smart Patients

https://www.smartpatients.com/

Appendix 2:
Selected Resources
for Whole Food
Plant-Based Diet

Dean Ornish, M.D. diet website:

https://www.ornish.com/proven-program/nutrition/

Michael Greger, M.D. website:

https://nutritionfacts.org/

T. Colin Campbell, Ph.D. website:

https://nutritionstudies.org/the-china-study/

Forks Over Knives website:

https://www.forksoverknives.com/our-story/

Physicians' Committee for Responsible Medicine website:

https://www.pcrm.org/

Appendix 3: Calcium Content of Foods from the USDA

Note: Most non-dairy plant milk is also calcium-rich—examine the nutrition label for details

Standard Portions

Calcium: Nutrient-dense[a] Food and Beverage Sources, Amounts of Calcium and Energy per Standard Portion

FOOD[bc]	STANDARD PORTION[d]	CALORIES	CALCIUM (mg)
Dairy and Fortified Soy Alternatives			
Yogurt, plain, nonfat	8 ounces	137	488
Yogurt, plain, low fat	8 ounces	154	448
Kefir, plain, low fat	1 cup	104	317
Milk, low fat (1%)	1 cup	102	305
Soy beverage (soy milk), unsweetened	1 cup	80	301
Yogurt, soy, plain	8 ounces	150	300
Milk, fat free (skim)	1 cup	83	298
Buttermilk, low fat	1 cup	98	284
Yogurt, Greek, plain, low fat	8 ounces	166	261
Yogurt, Greek, plain, nonfat	8 ounces	134	250
Cheese, reduced, low, or fat free (various)	1 ½ ounces	~55–155	~115–485
Vegetables			
Lambsquarters, cooked	1 cup	58	464
Nettles, cooked	1 cup	37	428
Mustard spinach, cooked	1 cup	29	284
Amaranth leaves, cooked	1 cup	28	276
Collard greens, cooked	1 cup	63	268
Spinach, cooked	1 cup	41	245

FOOD[bc]	STANDARD PORTION[d]	CALORIES	CALCIUM (mg)
Nopales, cooked	1 cup	22	244
Taro root (dasheen or yautia), cooked	1 cup	60	204
Turnip greens, cooked	1 cup	29	197
Bok choy, cooked	1 cup	24	185
Jute, cooked	1 cup	32	184
Kale, cooked	1 cup	43	177
Mustard greens, cooked	1 cup	36	165
Beet greens, cooked	1 cup	39	164
Pak choi, cooked	1 cup	20	158
Dandelion greens, cooked	1 cup	35	147
Protein Foods[e]			
Tofu, raw, regular, prepared with calcium sulfate	½ cup	94	434
Sardines, canned	3 ounces	177	325
Salmon, canned, solids with bone	3 ounces	118	181
Tahini (seasame butter or paste)	1 tablespoon	94	154
Fruit			
Grapefruit juice, 100%, fortified	1 cup	94	350
Orange juice, 100%, fortified	1 cup	117	349
Other Sources			
Almond beverage (almond milk), unsweetened	1 cup	36	442
Rice beverage (rice milk), unsweetened	1 cup	113	283

Smaller Portions

Calcium: Nutrient-dense[a] Food and Beverage Sources, Amounts of Calcium and Energy per Smaller Portion

FOOD[bc]	SMALLER PORTION[d]	CALORIES	CALCIUM (mg)
Dairy and Fortified Soy Alternatives			
Yogurt, plain, nonfat	4 ounces	69	244
Yogurt, plain, low fat	4 ounces	77	224
Kefir, plain, low fat	½ cup	52	159
Milk, low fat (1 %)	½ cup	51	153
Soy beverage (soy milk), unsweetened	½ cup	40	151
Yogurt, soy, plain	4 ounces	75	150
Milk, fat free (skim)	½ cup	42	149
Buttermilk, low fat	½ cup	49	142
Yogurt, Greek, plain, low fat	4 ounces	83	131
Yogurt, Greek, plain, nonfat	4 ounces	67	125
Cheese, reduced, low, or fat free (various)	½ ounce	~20-50	~40-160
Vegetables			
Lambsquarters, cooked	½ cup	29	232
Nettles, cooked	½ cup	19	214
Mustard spinach, cooked	½ cup	15	142
Amaranth leaves, cooked	½ cup	14	138
Collard greens, cooked	½ cup	32	134
Spinach, cooked	½ cup	21	123
Nopales, cooked	½ cup	11	122
Taro root (dasheen or yautia), cooked	½ cup	30	102

FOOD[bc]	SMALLER PORTION[d]	CALORIES	CALCIUM (mg)
Turnip greens, cooked	½ cup	15	99
Bok choy, cooked	½ cup	12	93
Jute, cooked	½ cup	16	92
Kale, cooked	½ cup	22	89
Mustard greens, cooked	½ cup	18	83
Beet greens, cooked	½ cup	20	82
Pak choi, cooked	½ cup	10	79
Dandelion greens, cooked	½ cup	18	74
Protein Foods[e]			
Tofu, raw, regular, prepared with calcium sulfate	¼ cup	47	217
Sardines, canned	1 ounce	59	108
Salmon, canned, solids with bone	1 ounce	39	60
Tahini (sesame butter or paste)	1 teaspoon	31	51
Fruit			
Grapefruit juice, 100%, fortified	½ cup	47	175
Orange juice, 100%, fortified	½ cup	59	175
Other Sources			
Almond beverage (almond milk), unsweetened	½ cup	18	221
Rice beverage (rice milk), unsweetened	½ cup	57	142

a All foods listed are assumed to be in nutrient-dense forms; lean or low-fat and prepared with minimal added sugars, saturated fat, or sodium.

b Some fortified foods and beverages are included. Other fortified options may exist on the market, but not all fortified foods are nutrient-dense. For example, some foods with added sugars may be fortified and would not be examples in the lists provided here.

c Some foods or beverages are not appropriate for all ages, particularly young children for whom some foods could be a choking hazard.

d Portions listed are not recommended serving sizes. Two lists—in 'standard' and 'smaller' portions--are provided for each dietary component. Standard portions provide at least 130 mg of calcium. Smaller portions are generally one half of a standard portion.

e Seafood varieties include choices from the FDA/EPA joint "Advice About Eating Fish," available at FDA.gov/fishadvice and EPA.gov/fishadvice from the "Best Choices" list. Varieties from the "Best Choices" list that contain even lower methylmercury include: flatfish (e.g., flounder), salmon, tilapia, shrimp, catfish, crab, trout, haddock, oysters, sardines, squid, pollock, anchovies, crawfish, mullet, scallops, whiting, clams, shad, and Atlantic mackerel.

Data Source: U.S. Department of Agriculture, Agricultural Research Service. FoodData Central, 2019. fdc.nal.usda.gov.

Notes

1 Rees F, Doherty M, Grainge MJ, Lanyon P, Zhang W. "The worldwide incidence and prevalence of systemic lupus erythematosus: a systematic review of epidemiological studies." Rheumatology (Oxford). 2017 Nov 1;56(11):1945-1961. DOI: 10.1093/rheumatology/kex260. PMID: 28968809.

2 Lima SC, Gomes da Silva IIF, Nascimento DQ, de Moura RR, Mesquita MDS, Asano NMJ, Fernandes GV, Valente LM, Rushansky E, Mariano MHQA, Xavier RM, Chies JAB, Crovella S, Sandrin-Garcia P. "CIITA gene polymorphism (rs3087456) in systemic lupus erythematosus and rheumatoid arthritis: A population-based cohort study." Int J Immunogenet. 2021 Oct;48(5):429-434. DOI: 10.1111/iji.12548. Epub 2021 Jun 27. PMID: 34180145.

3 Medina-Quiñones CV, Ramos-Merino L, Ruiz-Sada P, Isenberg D. "Analysis of Complete Remission in Systemic Lupus Erythematosus Patients Over a 32-Year Period. Arthritis Care Res (Hoboken). 2016 Jul;68(7):981-7. DOI: 10.1002/acr.22774. PMID: 26554745.

4 Sinski, C., Colligan, L., et al. "Allocation of physician time in ambulatory practice." Ann. Intern. Med. 2016;165-753-760.

5 Aguirre A, Izadi Z, Trupin L, Barbour KE, Greenlund KJ, Katz P, Lanata C, Criswell L, Dall'Era M, Yazdany J. "Race, Ethnicity, and Disparities

in the Risk of End-Organ Lupus Manifestations Following a Systemic Lupus Erythematosus Diagnosis in a Multiethnic Cohort." Arthritis Care Res (Hoboken). 2022 Apr 22. DOI: 10.1002/acr.24892. Epub ahead of print. PMID: 35452566.

6   https://www.lupusuk.org.uk/member-survey-results/

7   Booth S, Price E, Walker E. "Fluctuation, invisibility, fatigue – the barriers to maintaining employment with systemic lupus erythematosus: results of an online survey." Lupus 2018; 27: 2284–2291.

8   Agarwal N, Kumar V. "Burden of lupus on work: Issues in the employment of individuals with lupus." Work. 2016 Oct 17;55(2):429-439. DOI: 10.3233/WOR-162398. PMID: 27689581.

9   Daly R, Al Sawah S, Foster S, et al. "Health-Related Quality of Life in Lupus Differs by How Patients Perceive their Health and How Often They Experience Flares: Findings from a Cross-Sectional Online Survey in the United States." Annals of the Rheumatic Diseases 2015;74:578-579. https://ard.bmj.com/content/74/Suppl_2/578.3 (accessed October 21, 2021).

10   Real, Terrence. *US: Getting Past You & Me to Build a More Loving Relationship.* Rodale Books, 2022.

11   O'Rourke, Meghan. *The Invisible Kingdom: Reimagining Chronic Illness.* Riverhead Books, March 2022.

12   Hamburg, M., Cohen, M., DeSalvo, K., et al. "Building a National Public Health System in the United States." New England J Medicine 387;5. Aug. 4, 2022.

13   https://www.commonwealthfund.org/press-release/2021/new-international-study-us-health-system-ranks-last-among-11-countries-many

14   Kirzinger et al., "Health Tracking Poll March 2022: Economic concerns and health policy, the ACA, and views of long-term care facilities," Kaiser Family Foundation, 3/31/2022.

15   https://www.healthcare.gov/health-care-law-protections/grand fathered-plans/

16   https://findanafc.org/home/pro-bono/

17   Sharif K, Watad A, Bragazzi NL, Lichtbroun M, Amital H, Shoenfeld Y. "Physical activity and autoimmune diseases: Get moving and manage

the disease." Autoimmun Rev. 2018 Jan;17(1):53-72. DOI: 10.1016/j. autrev.2017.11.010. Epub 2017 Nov 3. PMID: 29108826.

18   Huston P, McFarlane B. "Health benefits of tai chi: What is the evidence?" Can Fam Physician. 2016 Nov;62(11):881-890. PMID: 28661865.

19   Ross A, Thomas S. "The health benefits of yoga and exercise: a review of comparison studies." J Altern Complement Med. 2010 Jan;16(1):3-12. DOI: 10.1089/acm.2009.0044. PMID: 20105062

20   https://www.youtube.com/watch?v=o8SjystaH-E&ab_channel= FishmanMethod

21   https://www.consumerreports.org/sunscreen/best-sunscreens-of-the-year-a7763432372/

22   WT, Ports TA, Kirkeeide RL, Hogeboom C, Brand RJ. "Intensive life-style changes for reversal of coronary heart disease." JAMA. 1998 Dec 16;280(23):2001-7. DOI: 10.1001/jama.280.23.2001. Erratum in: JAMA 1999 Apr 21;281(15):1380. PMID: 9863851.

23   Daly R, Al Sawah S, Foster S, et al. "Health-Related Quality of Life in Lupus Differs by How Patients Perceive their Health and How Often They Experience Flares: Findings from a Cross-Sectional Online Survey in the United States." Annals of the Rheumatic Diseases 2015;74:578-579. https://ard.bmj.com/content/74/Suppl_2/578.3 (accessed October 21, 2021).

24   Knippenberg A, Robinson GA, Wincup C, Ciurtin C, Jury EC, Kalea AZ. "Plant-based dietary changes may improve symptoms in patients with systemic lupus erythematosus." Lupus. 2022 Jan;31(1):65-76. DOI: 10.1177/09612033211063795. Epub 2022 Jan 3. PMID: 34978516; PMCID:

25   Sanches MS, Rodrigues da Silva C, Silva LC, Montini VH, Lopes Barboza MG, Migliorini Guidone GH, Dias de Oliva BH, Nishio EK, Faccin Galhardi LC, Vespero EC, Lelles Nogueira MC, Dejato Rocha SP. "Proteus mirabilis from community-acquired urinary tract infections (UTI-CA) shares genetic similarity and virulence factors with isolates from chicken, beef and pork meat." Microb Pathog. 2021 Sep; 158:105098. DOI: 10.1016/j.micpath.2021.105098. Epub 2021 Jul 17. PMID: 34280499.

26 Buberg ML, Mo SS, Sekse C, Sunde M, Wasteson Y, Witsø IL. Population structure and uropathogenic potential of extended-spectrum cephalosporin-resistant Escherichia coli from retail chicken meat. BMC Microbiol. 2021 Mar 29;21(1):94. DOI: 10.1186/s12866-021-02160-y. PMID: 33781204; PMCID: PMC8008618.

27 https://www.hopkinslupus.org/lupus-info/lifestyle-additional-information/avoid/

28 Harrison SR, Li D, Jeffery LE, Raza K, Hewison M. Vitamin D, Autoimmune Disease and Rheumatoid Arthritis. Calcif Tissue Int. 2020 Jan;106(1):58-75. DOI: 10.1007/s00223-019-00577-2. Epub 2019 Jul 8. PMID: 31286174; PMCID: PMC6960236.

29 LeBoff MS, Chou SH, Ratliff KA, Cook NR, Khurana B, Kim E, Cawthon PM, Bauer DC, Black D, Gallagher JC, Lee IM, Buring JE, Manson JE. Supplemental Vitamin D and Incident Fractures in Midlife and Older Adults. N Engl J Med. 2022 Jul 28;387(4):299-309. DOI: 10.1056/NEJMoa2202106. PMID: 35939577

30 Parisis D, Bernier C, Chasset F, Arnaud L. Impact of tobacco smoking upon disease risk, activity and therapeutic response in systemic lupus erythematosus: A systematic review and meta-analysis. Autoimmun Rev. 2019 Nov;18(11):102393. DOI: 10.1016/j.autrev.2019.102393. Epub 2019 Sep 11. PMID: 31520802.

31 Gayed M, Bernatsky S, Ramsey-Goldman R, Clarke A, Gordon C. "Lupus and cancer." Lupus. 2009 May;18(6):479-85. DOI: 10.1177/0961203309102556. PMID: 19395448.

32 Costedoat-Chalumeau N, Dunogué B, Morel N, Le Guern V, Guettrot-Imbert G. "Hydroxychloroquine: a multifaceted treatment in lupus." Presse Med. 2014 Jun;43(6 Pt 2):e167-80. DOI: 10.1016/j.lpm.2014.03.007. Epub 2014 May 19. PMID: 24855048.

33 https://www.hopkinslupus.org/lupus-info/lifestyle-additional-information/avoid/

34 Cocco F, Carta G, Cagetti MG, Strohmenger L, Lingström P, Campus G. "The caries preventive effect of 1-year use of low-dose xylitol chewing gum. A randomized placebo-controlled clinical trial in high-caries-risk adults." Clin Oral Investig. 2017 Dec; 21(9):2733-2740.

35 Darcey J, Horner K, Walsh T, Southern H, Marjanovic EJ, Devlin H. "Tooth loss and osteoporosis: to assess the association between osteoporosis status and tooth number." Br Dent J. 2013 Feb;214(4): E10. DOI: 10.1038/sj.bdj.2013.165. PMID: 23429157.

36 Vitlic A, Lord JM, Phillips AC. "Stress, ageing and their influence on functional, cellular and molecular aspects of the immune system." Age (Dordr). 2014 Jun;36(3):9631. DOI: 10.1007/s11357-014-9631-6. Epub 2014 Feb 25. PMID: 24562499; PMCID: PMC4082590.

37 Moyers, Bill. *Healing and the Mind.* Doubleday, 1993.

38 Mueller PS, Plevak DJ, Rummans TA. "Religious involvement, spirituality, and medicine: implications for clinical practice." Mayo Clin Proc. 2001 Dec;76(12):1225-35. DOI: 10.4065/76.12.1225. PMID: 11761504.

39 https://news.harvard.edu/gazette/story/2017/04/over-nearly-80-years-harvard-study-has-been-showing-how-to-live-a-healthy-and-happy-life/

40 Lawton, R.N., Gramatki, I., Watt, W. *et al.* "Does Volunteering Make Us Happier, or Are Happier People More Likely to Volunteer? Addressing the Problem of Reverse Causality When Estimating the Wellbeing Impacts of Volunteering." *J Happiness Stud* 22, 599–624 (2021). https://doi.org/10.1007/s10902-020-00242-8

41 https://www.coursera.org/learn/the-science-of-well-being

42 https://www.psychologytoday.com/us/blog/resilience/202208/there-is-no-formula-happiness

www.ingramcontent.com/pod-product-compliance
Lightning Source LLC
Chambersburg PA
CBHW060514130626

46553CB00002B/485